CONTENTS

PREFACE

What is Yoga

Any more or less educated person has heard about yoga. But if you ask what is yoga, you will have a wide range of various and often contradictory definitions: from «Indian gymnastics» to «religious philosophic teaching», from «fakir art» to «system of spiritual perfection», from «relic of ancient civilizations» to a «gift of extraterrestrial intelligence». More «competent» interlocutor will also recall about Buddhist yoga (the less competent can confuse Buddhism with yoga), Taoist yoga and many others. Speaking about yoga we also think about Tantra, which an uneducated interlocutor can call «the yoga of sex».

So what is yoga? Is it a purely Indian phenomena or does it go through different world traditions, as many people think? How ancient is this teaching? Is it a canonic learning transmitted from generation to generation or is it a dynamic developing system? Or maybe it is just a reconstructed tradition like the «classical» Indian dance Bharatnatyam, invented only in XIX century or the animal kung fu fighting, contrived by the Institute of Physical Culture in Beijing? Can we really define «Chinese», «Russian» or «modern» yoga? After all is yoga a religion? If not, why is it so often confused with it? Let's try to give preliminary answers to these questions.

In every culture and religion there traditionally was a specific system, mainly practical, used by the limited number of disciples. Such systems are called esoteric (from the Greek «inward»). For example, Sufism was such a system within Islam, Hesychasm within Orthodoxy, Neydan within Taosism, Spiritual Exercises of Ignatius of Loyola in Catholisism etc. Esoteric systems are hidden deep inside of religions and fundamentally differ from them. First of all by the fact that... they are not religions. Actually what makes them special and «secret» is that unlike religion esoteric systems they are highly practical. They have the same goal as religions: to make **personality consciously change**, but unlike religions these systems offer a defined set of methods to make such changes. Those changes are based on the changed state of mind. But unlike religionists, followers of esoteric systems strive for long-lasting changes of personality.

11

If you compare objects and values of religions and their esoteric systems, you'll see some clear distinctions, although they are not much proclaimed.

The reader might already see what I'm getting at. Yoga is an esoteric system within Indian tradition. Only Indian? Is there any rapport between different esoteric systems? Are they all independent or did they evolve one from another? Or maybe they all evolved from one more ancient unknown system? Or is this more ancient system yoga itself? After all it is the most ancient of all esoteric systems. Indeed comparing practices of different esoteric systems you'll find many obvious analogies. For example, if you read one of the Hesychasm classics Gregory Palamas, who suggests to inhale the «red air» by one nostril and to exhale the «blue air» with another, if you are somewhat familiar with yoga you would exclaim: «Hey, it's Anuloma Viloma! They happened to know about Ida and Pingala». It might seem an obvious adoption, but is it? Is it because of the same object of influence — man and his psyche? Did different esoteric systems come to the same techniques, because they were the most effective?

Tracing back the history of yoga we meet with some difficulties. Although we can find terms «yoga» and «yogin» in the Mahabharata so that they obviously date before the Vedic period, the activity they meant often differs a lot from what we call yoga now. Furthermore even then there have already been discords in definition of yoga. Everyone agreed upon two thinks: a) yoga is a system of methods and b) yoga is a secret (esoteric) system. Analyzing ancient scripts you will also find evidence that yoga **had a common object, which was to change ontological status of the practitioner in the world**. Overlooking other esoteric systems we'll easily see that they had the same goals. Taoists grow the spiritual germ, Hesychasts strive for an «angel rank in this life», Buddhists seek for Enlightenment etc. Is it an adoption? Or is it once more the same object?

We can try to track down how yoga was forming. We'll find Aryan and Dravidian background, find parallels with Shaman practices, Matriarchal cults, primitive magic and so on. We can track the origin of yoga back to the prehistoric civilizations, although it goes beyond the scope of this book. It is exiting and edifying. But probably the reader has already got my attitude to this subject. We can never find precise answers to all our questions, and it doesn't really matter. Above all I hope we»ve already understood: **the idea of the Way, the spiritual evolution is archetypical**. This way or another it always comes to any tradition whether it is prehistoric culture, religious system or materialistic soviet culture. The unity of yoga is not in details and historic references. **Yoga is common in its spirit.** That is why despite all persecutions it still exists and survived most of its «persecutors».

Does the line of authority exist in yoga transmission? Is there such thing as «classic» yoga? I don't think so. Such a view reminds me the times we were kids and believed in wise old guys who have all the answers, you just have to ask them well... Besides such a point of view is philosophically inconsistent. Where would those «guys» get that knowledge? Should we refer to extraterrestrials? Then how did they invent yoga?

No, at the heart of any esoteric tradition stand some real people, who by an inconceivable act of spiritual enlightenment have seen further than others. Sometimes their disciples kept their teaching on, climbing higher and higher, although more often they just used this teaching or turned it into a cult. Many great teachings degenerated into religions. Unfortunately it's much easier to worship than to think and to create...

Esoteric knowledge has another distinctive feature. It cannot be transmitted without personal practice. It is «hidden» not just because someone is hiding it (although it's also true) — you can't conceive it without making radical changes in yourself. **Esoteric knowledge cannot be KNOWN. It can only be LIVED.** Otherwise it makes no sense. The understanding of every new level is possible only after the previous one is passed. It is not an act of learning, but our personal mystical experience. Esoteric knowledge cannot be transmitted in a form of scripts and tables. It must be given from the teacher to a student. The Teacher must have patience and wish to lighten fire of spirit in his student, and the student must be ready and willing to become a co-creator of himself. A Chinese martial tradition has a saying: «There is no style — just Master's personal technique». Restating this maxim we can say: «There is no classic yoga — just Teacher's personal yoga». It works in his hands and helps his students to change and to create their own Yoga, which stops being yoga, a method, if canonized. An esoteric teaching is inseparable from its bearer and its Teacher. While only Life can prove, if the teaching is effective and right.

Did objects and methods of yoga change through the centuries of its existence? The answer comes logically from the aforesaid: yes, constantly. But in details. Different times and different people need different words and methods. But the said above object is always there. The changing of a status can also be different. As well as the levels of Teachers.

So **yoga is not a religion**. Living «here and now» is not less important for a yogi than his spiritual tasks. That is why along with the Big Yoga, setting its higher aims there's always been the Small Yoga — a system of methods (once again — methods), aimed at life improvement: health, wealth, emotional state. At that the Small Yoga practice is not a diversion from the Spiritual Way, but its essential element.

Yoga is not a practice of asceticism. For a harmonic and creative existence you need to love life. Although elements of ascetic practices can be used as one of the methods.

Yoga is not a philosophy, but it has philosophic basics and methods based on philosophic practice. Over years yoga repeatedly changed its philosophies (plural), explaining the same practices in different words.

Yoga is not an ethic system. Every ethic system is in the long run engendered by the religious perception of the world, by the fear of punishment, by the supreme forces etc. Yoga has its rules too (*Yama*, for example), which can be mistaken for ethical, but their essence is principally different. Yogi follows these rules not because he is afraid of punishment — it is his most pragmatic choice allowing him to save energy as much as possible. On the higher levels all rules disappear and give way to the principles.

Understanding of **principles** is the primary perceptive object of yoga. The comprehension of yoga principles is the objective of this book.

Hatha in the system of Yoga

All the methods of Hatha Yoga are meant for gaining success in the Raja-Yoga.

Hatha Yoga Pradipika

Practically in every esoteric teaching there was a special system assigned to work with the physical body — one of the differences between esotericism and religion. Gymnastics of Hermes, wushu, styles of Qigong, whirling dervishes, Zikri, Zongshen — the gymnastics[1] of Vietnamese monachs, breathing practices of Hesychasts and so on. Although the most developed and sophisticated, as well as probably the most ancient of them is Hatha yoga.

What is the sense of work with the physical body within an esoteric tradition? Just to strengthen it in order to prepare for more difficult psychical exercises? Maybe, but then you don't need such refined exercises. The ordinary gymnastics, invented by Greeks (almost all nations had its analogues), perfectly strengthens our body. Healing the body? Indeed yoga has its therapeutic effect, but not as a chief aim. Already many centuries ago yoga was said to be for strong and healthy people. Not to mention that medical treatment (Tibetan medicine) gives outstanding results and demands from patient much less efforts. Maybe its objective is to attain extraordinary physical capacities: force, flexibility, stamina? Nonsense, of course, if you are not going to make a career as a circus acrobat… Then what is the sense of physical training within esoteric traditions? What is the most important for us, what is the sense of Hatha?

To answer this question let's remember that yoga is a system, aimed at the conscious changing of a person, at the self-change, conscious restructuring of our psyche, of our subtle bodies. But human's psyche is difficult to study — to say nothing about our subtle bodies, even more difficult to work with, because a common person cannot see them. This is when we can use the connection between our physical body and our subtle bodies along with our psyche. Our physical body becomes a clue to all the processes that take place in our subtler bodies.

---

[1]   I conventionally call it «gymnastics», for the lack of more appropriate term. In fact all the listed techniques are fundamentally differ (even in the way of looking) from what Greeks used to call «gymnastics».

Indeed our physical body is the reflection of our subtle bodies. Whatever is below is similar to that which is above. But unlike subtle bodies, our physical body can be touched and seen. All processes happening in our subtle bodies are reflected in our physical body. So that all possible problems of our psyche, of our ether and astral bodies are reflected in the *stature* of our physical body in the form of physical constraints: contractions, curvatures of the spine — they show our state of chakral system and in the limit — our diseases[1].

The contrary is also true: by influencing our body, we influence our psyche. That's what Hatha is about, that was its place and objective in the system of Yoga.

Do the objectives of yoga change? I think we can definitely answer «yes». Psychologically a modern European is completely different from a Hindu. We are people «living by our head», while Hindu were to greater extent sensitive, living mostly by their feelings and emotions. This makes our ways to the spiritual harmony different: for Hindu this way had to do with the «lifting» the energy (here's where *Kundalini* comes from), while for us it is putting it down, developing our physical sensitivity.

That is why using Indian practices automatically, without adapting them to our modern cultural and historic conditions is a false way, leading away from the harmony and turning yoga itself — an exceptionally rational and pragmatic system — into a religion.

HUMAN ENERGY STRUCTURE

Energy bodies

Nearly all esoteric systems believe that a person, beside a physical body, has the so-called «fine» bodies: seven bodies, four of which are the brightest, while the others remain so fine that it is hard to notice them in our everyday life.

Etheric body (Sanskrit: *Prana Kosha*, sheath made of prana) in other schools also called vital body, which **defines the structure of human health**. If you have a cut or a scratch, ultimately your skin heals –regeneration program is defined by our etheric body. The stronger it is, the healthier you are, and the weaker, the more valetudinarian you are. The etheric body has the form of our physical body. There is also an **etheric field**. It's our etheric energy, not structured in the etheric body and surrounding us as a bag of 0.4–1 m (for the healthy person). Etheric field stands in a dynamic balance with the etheric body. Our etheric body rarely changes its form, normally when we become seriously ill. When we have a lot of energy: we ate a lot, energetically nibbled someone (it also happens), stayed in some places with a lot of etheric energy, all the extra energy goes to the etheric field, making it bigger. In special cases etheric field can widen up to 1,5–2 meters, it can be very big, but not for a long time. If someone has a lot of etheric field energy, ultimately he'll be «eaten around», because one cannot carry along a lot of energy. When we speak about human aura and the size of its field, we mean **etheric field**.

Only living objects, including minerals, have **an etheric field**. By definition it's a non-physical field, so any attempts to measure it by physical devices are insensate. It can only be measured by devices using living objects: germs, plants, animals, people and their reaction on the energy. The most common way of measuring etheric field is biolocation. The etheric field as well as the etheric body can be seen on the homogeneous background, but it is more rarefied.

Astral body (Sanskrit: *Koma Kosha* — sheath of desires) defines the structure of our etheric body. If etheric body destabilises, the astral body gives a regeneration program. Astral body repeats the outline of our etheric and physical bodies and is situated outside the etheric body. It also can be seen on the homogeneous background.

Astral body defines our emotional state. Astral field is a volume of the astral energy, which is in dynamic balance with the astral body. If we say: «What a charismatic person!» we react on an astral field. A person with a strong astral field can influence other peoples' emotions. Sociology and psychology call it charisma. Being close to such a person it's easy to get involved in his emotional state.

To feel astral energies one needs no special skills. In the society you feel that the ambience is distressing, at this point you»ve switched to the feeling of astral energies of this company. If you feel that the atmosphere is joyful and you have fun, you're feeling these energies this way. **The capacity to switch to surrounding astral energies and getting these states on the conscious level is the «exiting to astral».**

Of course astral fields cannot be measured by physical instruments either.

Mental body (Sanskrit: *Mana Kosha* — sheath of mind, manasa) is ideas, thoughts, knowledge, and senses.

Discussion of higher planes and fields is above the theme of this book.

Human's Chakral System

History

The main element of human energy structure is chakral system. Chakras (Sanskrit: *Chakra* — wheel or disc) are mentioned in the most part of Yoga and Tantra origins, such as «Gheranda samhita», «Hatha Yoga Pradipika», «Shiva samhita», «Shat Chakra nirupane», «Yoga Tattva Upanishada», «Amritabindu Upanishada» and many others (see Appendix 2).

Chakras are also mentioned in Tibetan origins such as in the famous Atlas of Tibetan medicine, in Chinese treatises of Neidan (Sanskrit: *neidan* — inner elixir). Some elements of chakral system are mentioned in Japanese martial arts (hara, ten-sho), in outlooks of Mesoamerican shamans. These notions are also met in less developed systems (naturally, in simplified version).

The Western world[1] learned about chakras thanks to the proceedings of Arthur Avalon, a European who got into the restricted Indian Tantric School and afterwards has published notions he received. He was the first to publish classical Indian drawings of chakras, which have been redrawn for last 100 years by other authors with all imagin-

---

[1]   General public. Alchemists and representatives of other esoteric systems in Europe has known about chakral system before.

able errors and distortions. He also gave mantras for chakras and their petals, correlated petals with human qualities. Based on his chakral scheme a countless number of schools and interpretations were born, as well as various techniques of work with chakras. Although being an adept of an esoteric school, Avalon made some hay of understanding chakral system, affirming that one can open chakras by «raising Kundalini», while an common person has all chakras closed.

The next step in understanding the chakral system in modern occult tradition was made by Rudolph Steiner, the founder of anthroposophist society. He noticed that chakras don't open while raising Kundalini, on the contrary: **people open their chakras, acquiring some qualities and skills,** which creates prerequisites for raising Kundalini. Thanks to Steiner's observation the concept of chakral system in modern esotericism has broadened. In Steiner's works he affirms that all people have chakras, but their level of development can differ. Moreover the chakra's characteristics define our actions, capacities and personality.

At the same time psychology also approached the problem of chakral system.

Wilhelm Reich further acknowledged as a founder of the body psychotherapy has found out that psychological problems lead to muscle blocks, localising as **seven** «muscle armours», each of them reflecting a certain well-defined group of problems. (I suppose, that even those readers who don't know about works of Reich have already guessed that position and characteristics of these «armours» amazingly reminded Steiner's chakral system). This theory was significantly developed by progenies and followers of Reich (A. Lowen, Feldenkreiz), while body-psychotherapy has taken a fare place among other therapeutic systems. The Western world was finding its first clues.

A certain input in understanding the chakral system and its role in studying human body was done by mediums in the period of great interest to the extrasensory capacities in the late 1970s. Mostly independently from the mentioned origins based on their personal experience, mediums noticed that human body has energy centres and a man's health depends on their state. These centres are located practically in the same place as Avalon's lotuses.

However no wonder all the systems independently were coming to the same conclusions. Chakras exist in reality and any studying of a human being ultimately leads to similar notions. The connection between emotional states and certain parts of body is also reflected in such metaphors as «to have a clear head», «a thick-headed person», «lump in one's throat», «a heart withered», «to be a pain in the neck», «a great weight off one's mind», «a sinking sensation in the pit of one's stomach», «ants in one's pants», «a pain in the ass».

Physiological aspects of chakras

Let's briefly describe the localisation and symbols of chakras according to the Indian tradition.

SAHASRARA is located in the crown of the head. Its exact symbol is unknown.

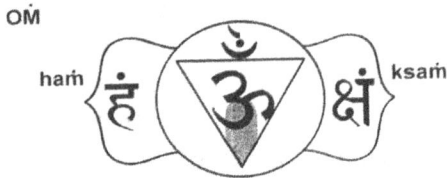

AJNA is located between eyebrows and relates to the pineal gland. Anatomically relates to the brain, eyes, frontal and maxillary sinuses, nose, and upper teeth.

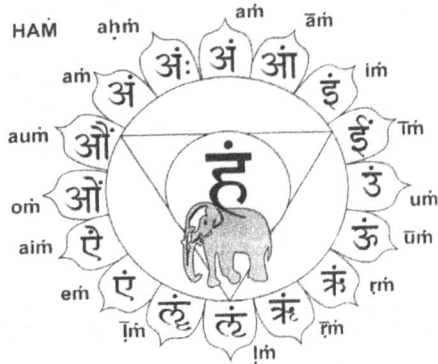

VISHUDDHA is located around the throat and relates to the thyroid and parathyroid gland, ears and everything in the larynx, with gullet, trachea, upper bronchus, tongue and cervical vertebra.

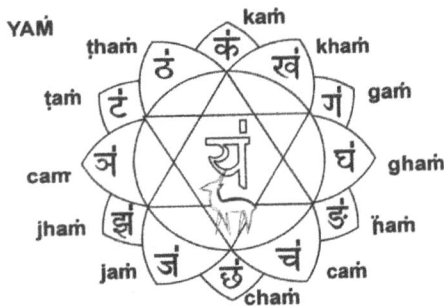

ANAHATA, a heart chakra. Controls cardiovascular system, mainly the heart itself, lungs, thoracic vertebra, arms, ribs and all intercostal spaces, inferior bronchus.

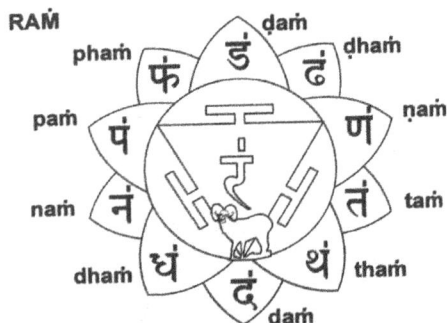

MANIPURA is located slightly over the navel and relates to the following organs: stomach, gastrointestinal tract (except the upper gullet), intestines, first of all with the small intestine (colon is more related to the Muladhara), upper kidneys and adrenals (adrenalin is a hormone of Manipura), liver, spleen, vertebra in the Manipura region, pancreas.

20

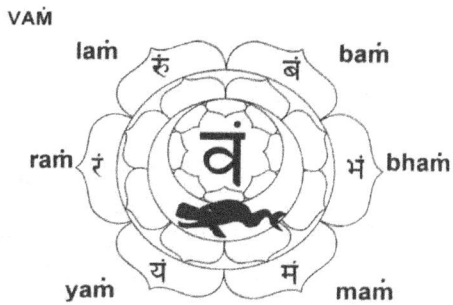

SVADHISTHANA is located in genitals, about 4 fingers down the navel. Related to the genitals (male and female), bladder, inferior kidneys, renal pelvises, ureters, uriniferous tubule (for women), lower back (except the sacrum, related to Muladhara), hips.

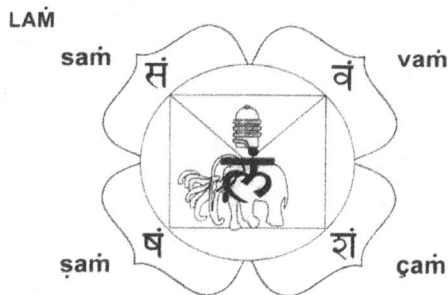

MULADHARA is located in the sacrum. It relates to the sacrum, prostate, pelvis, colon, rectum.

Chakras exist on the astral, etheric and physical planes. Correlating their localisation with endocrine glands and with the knots of autonomic nervous system (ANS) we can easily see the perfect analogy. This connection is absolute most of all, if you take into account additional chakras (4 for each primary chakra), mentioned in the Atlas of Tibetan Medicine. Physically every chakra is presented by a gland or an ANS node.

Nevertheless people are not just physics. That is why the chakral system is not limited by the particularities of our physical body. Chakra's characteristics are directly related to the human energy and psyche. As a matter of fact chakras are «a bridge», connecting our physical, etheric and astral bodies.

Psychological aspects of chakras

Chakra is a complicated notion with many parameters. They are often described from just one point of view. For example, saying it's strong or weak. Actually to describe chakra you need at least ten different parameters. Some of them are given below.

Chakra's strength

Chakra's strength is a volume of energy, initially present in a chakra, while its weakness is the absence of this energy. The energy in chakra determines our desires, and the more energy we have, the stronger our desires are. This fact explains the esoteric principle; **if you listen to your real desires, you follow your dharma.**

21

PICTURE 1. Endocrine glands

1 — pineal gland; 2 — epiphysis;
3 — pituitary gland;
4 — parathyroid gland;
5 — thyroid gland;
6 — thymus; 7 — pancreas;
8 — adrenal gland;
9 — ovary; 10 — testis.

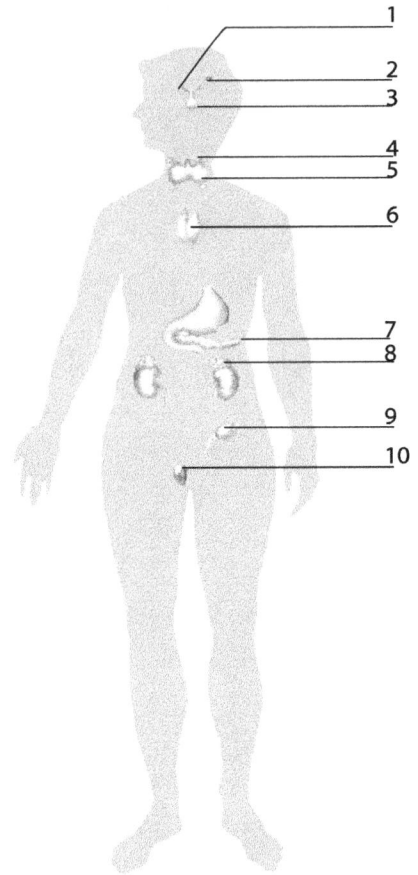

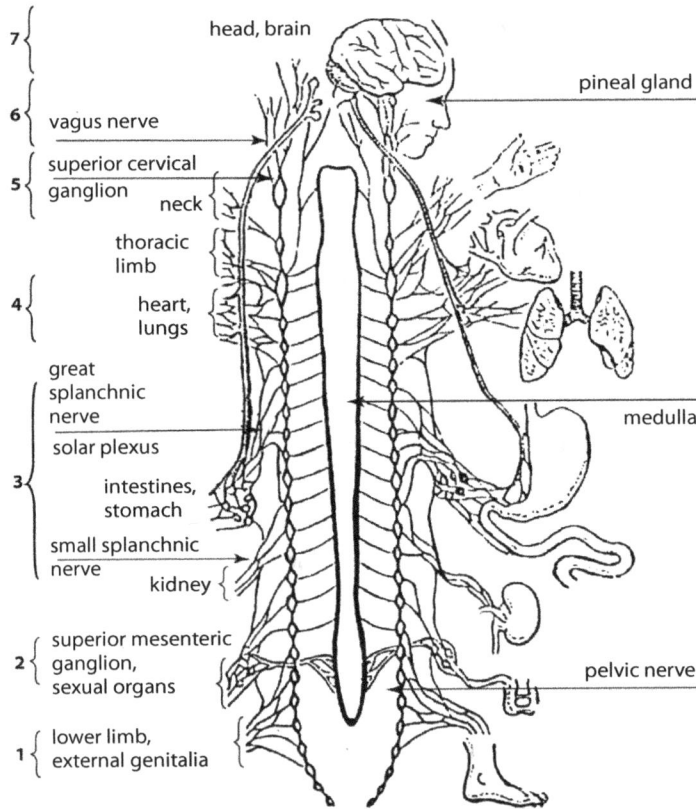

head, brain

pineal gland

7

6 vagus nerve

superior cervical
5 ganglion
neck

thoracic
limb

4 heart,
lungs

great
splanchnic
nerve

solar plexus

3 intestines,
stomach

small splanchnic
nerve
kidney

medulla

superior mesenteric
2 ganglion,
sexual organs

pelvic nerve

1 lower limb,
external genitalia

**PICTURE 2. Ganglia of ANS
and their correlation with
chakras**

From all above said it is easy to understand that a person with a strong chakra is highly motivated by needs related to this chakra; so we can make a psychological portrait of people with different strong chakras. For instance a person with strong Muladhara works for prosperity, routinely organizes his private space and is never tired of it. He likes it because it corresponds his needs and desires. Wherever he goes, he'll always put everything around in order — for better for worse. A person with a strong Muladhara doesn't like discomfort.

22

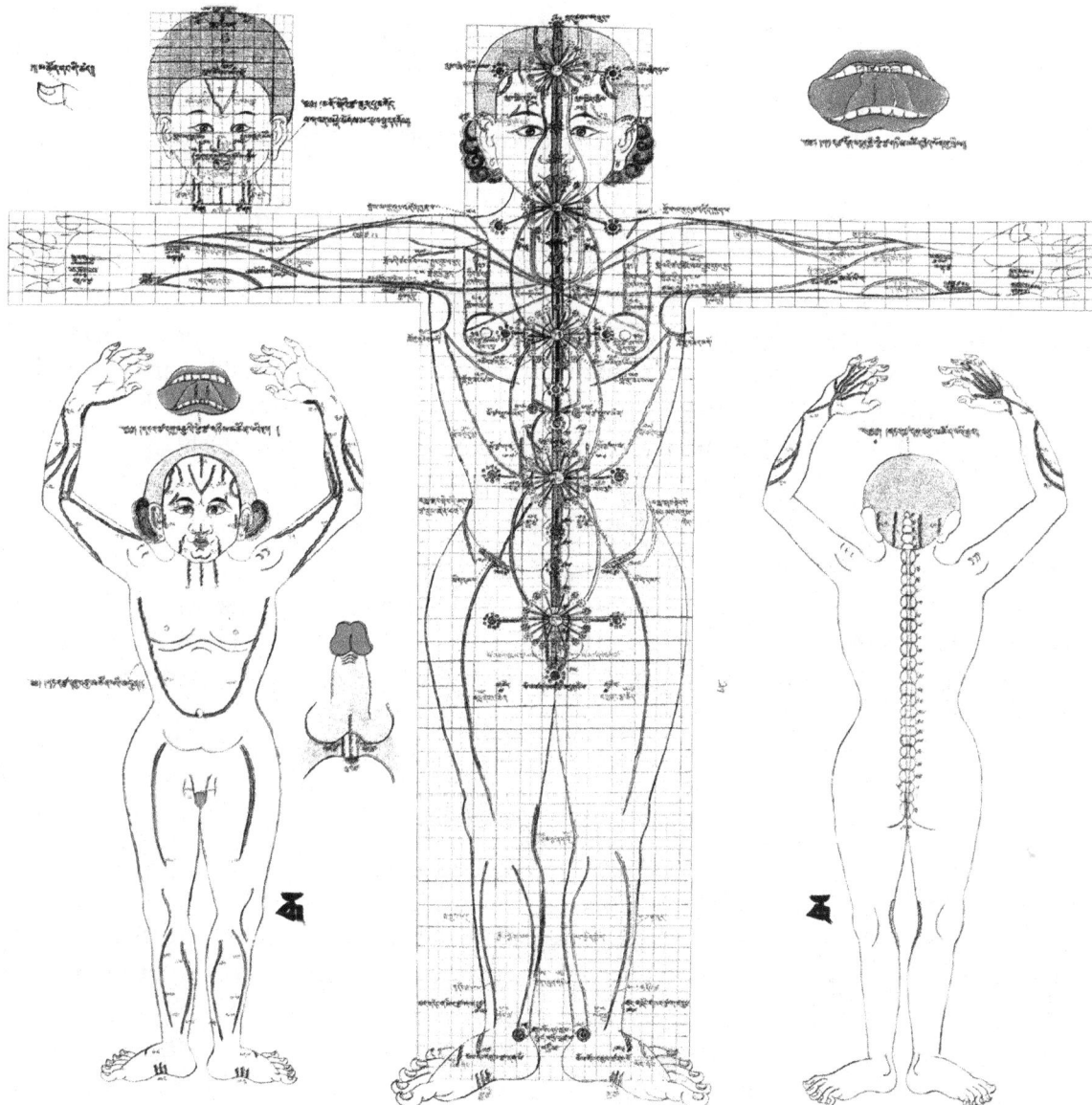

PICTURE 3. Figure of chakras from the «Atlas of Tibetan medicine»

The figure is interesting in a way that it marks not only the essential but also auxiliary chakras. It should be borne in mind that the Tibetans considered muladhara an auxiliary chakra

For a person with a strong **Svadhisthana** pleasures are one of the dominating motives. He looks for pleasure in everything, and, if he doesn't find it, he creates it. A motive of sensual pleasure, including sexual, is dominating for him.

A person with a strong **Manipura** is motivated by needs in dominating, governing, social recognition and respect. Such people live for their career.

A person with a strong **Anahata** lives with his feelings. For example, he or she can sacrifice something for love (or hatred which is just another feeling).

A person with a strong **Vishuddha** is motivated by perception of the World and his need to express himself. He or she is curious, inquisitive and often aesthetic. Vishuddha is also responsible for verbal intellect, i.e. the capacity to express one's thoughts in words.

A person with a strong **Ajna** is motivated by existential needs, i.e. a need to form his worldview, to see his place in the world, to understand the sense of life.

The upper chakra, **Sahasrara** and its characteristics are not studied in this book, because its expression has to do with the contact of a man and the Cosmos, Superior Powers and for most people is not so important.

Maturity of chakra.
Openness and closeness of chakra

First of all we should speak not about chakra's openness, but about its maturity or immaturity. **A mature chakra means a person has a lot of experience on it.**

The mature **Ajna** depending on it's development can allot a person observation skills, logical thinking, erudition, analytical thinking and deep wisdom.

If a person has a mature **Vishuddha**, he can verbally express his thoughts and feelings — in words or by other meanings.

Having a mature **Anahata** one knows how to operate with the energy of feelings. He can show his feelings and accepts those of others. He can be outstanding in emotional, sensitive sphere. Usually people with mature Anahata are very artistic.

A person with the mature **Manipura** is a person with the powerful social intelligence, meaning he's bellicose, independent, knows how to achieve his goals by socially accepted means, even to the prejudice of others.

A person with the mature **Svadhisthana** knows how to live with pleasure. He can get pleasure from life and give it to others. His pleasures are well defined, he's an expert in sophisticated delights and states.

A person with the mature **Muladhara** easily structures all around. Such people build many things, do repairs and put everything around them in order.

It can be that a person has a strong, but immature chakra.

Let's take for example, **Svadhisthana**. One can have a strong Svadhisthana with a lot of energy in it, but all the scope of his sensual delights is to eat, to drink and to sleep... In this case we say that chakra is strong, but immature.

The same with strong, but immature **Manipura**. It makes a person have tendency to dominate, but it's expressed in primitive forms: to beat someone, to humiliate, to scare. A person with such Manipura doesn't understand that there are subtler ways to dominate, more sophisticated forms of managing people, and, consequently, cannot use these means.

A person with a strong, but immature **Anahata** is overwhelmed with feelings, but he doesn't know what they are, he cannot neither express nor define his state.

A strong, but immature **Vishuddha** give rise to «inventors» of perpetual motion machines, amateur art activists and so on.

Thus every centre isn't just a drawing or a lotus on our backbone opening when Kundalini passes by. It is a well-defined set of psychic functions, expressing in everyday life like skills, abilities, capacities and qualities. Hence it is obvious that a person with mature chakras is more complete, than the one who has some unopened chakras.

The most usual, clear and natural combination is **a weak and immature chakra.** Such person hardly expresses himself on this chakra. Quite positive is a situation when a chakra is strong, but immature. Then he has a lot of energy and can afford himself to make mistakes and make some new experience. If he makes it his aim, he can develop his chakra. At that time he'll have less energy in it, because by the cut and try method he'll stumble many times and pay with his energy for new experience.

The more mature is chakra, the less energy you have to apply to achieve your goals related to this chakra.

Let's take the example of **Vishuddha**. Everyone needs a certain number of words to explain his thought to other people. The less this chakra is developed, the more words you need. One can explain for hours, another needs just a few words and bright images. Not only comprehensiveness, but also capacious ness of the speech is growing with Vishuddha's development. For example, Patanjali's «Sutra Yoga» is just four pages that can be interpreted and reinterpreted, because it is laconic. Information is so to say compact. Short phrases contain many meanings and nuances.

If a mature person «emanates» his energy of **Svadhisthana**, people around fall into a «high» state. If one uses energy of **Manipura**, others start feeling anxiety and fear. You can hardly approach such a person without a trepidation, and even a thought of attacking him scares you (for real). The more mature is chakra, the less energy a person needs having more ways to achieve his goals.

The openness of chakra is the ability to emanate energy directly, escaping any action. So a person with the open Vishuddha doesn't need words to explain. You come to ask him a question and suddenly you realise that you already know the answer. The ability to transmit your state and to express your feelings without speaking is a sign of an open Anahata and so on.

The openness of chakra is the attribute of yogin state. We call yogin a person who has opened all 7 chakras and is capable to emanate energy from each of them with no action.

Of course all the described states are *siddhas* — extra capacities, beyond «normal» or better to say usual human's abilities. **The capacity to manage outer etheric or astral field of any chakra is a siddha.** Opening any chakra we get a certain set of siddhas, while, if you don't have certain siddhas, it means your respective chakra is closed.

It's important to understand that not only those, who do occult practices can have siddhas. Common people often have some of these siddhas and very powerful ones, but they ignore their energy side. Realisation in society directly depends on siddhas he has. For example, can a person become a chief, if he doesn't make employees tremble by his only look? Does a doctor always understand why he makes such a diagnosis? Why one musician deeply affects listeners to tears, while another plays the same music just doing an accurate technique? The answer to these questions lies in the ability to work with energy.

Sometimes people use their siddhas unconsciously. Some do it semiconsciously. They know what to do, which state to take in order to make things happen, but there is a certain difference between a common person with some siddhas and an esoteric. A person in the society realises his skills, i.e. uses what he already has. The one who practices esotericism or yoga has a wider task. He tries not just to realise his abilities (which is also very important), but also to work out new capacities and skills to crucially change something in his life or in himself. This is what is called the work on opening our chakral system.

Energy channels

Ida and Pingala

«Hatha Yoga Pradipika» and other classical treatises assert that human being has 72 000 energy channels, but the most important and mentioned are 13, from which the primary three are: *Ida*, *Pingala* and *Sushumna*.

From the drawings we can easily see that chakras are located on the crossings (or better said interlacements) of ida and pingala. It is so, and chakras are formed by the crossings of these channels. The relative activity of chakra, its radiating and absorbing capacities depend on the current stage of our biological rhythm.

Ida and Pingala, so-called Sun and Moon channels, start on the right and left petals of Ajna and go down as showed at the picture. Moreover Ida is related to the right nostril and Pingala — to the left one. According to «Svaradoya shastra» the channel is active when the related nostril is open, i.e. when it's easier to breathe with. When a right nostril is active dissimulation processes prevail and as a result we have a burst of energy and become active (that is why it is called Sun channel). When Pingala is active, processes of assimilation prevail: the body is building itself, energy is absorbed and we want to rest and relax. Obviously Ida and Pingala consequently relate with the sympathetic and parasympathetic nervous systems.

It's interesting that this scheme, described in ancient Indian treatises, looks a lot like contemporary understandings about nervous system. Here is an extract from the description done by academician Smirnov: «The association with inner organs is done in two ways. The first is ascending and another — a descending way of white substance, of medulla with its segmental apparatus of grey matter, where parts are joint on the principle of series active components (Sushumna — A.S.). The second way — by the chain of boundary trunk of vegetative nervous system. The boundary trunk goes on the side of vertebra as a set of nodes, formed by a nerve cells accumulation; these nodes are connected in both directions by passers. A boundary trunk is a paired formation. Latest research of Ognev and his school has shown that the right and the left part of the trunk (Ida and Pingala — A. S.[1]) are not equipollent, how it was thought; the right and the left trunks fulfil similar, but not identical functions: the left one is responsible for arterial vasomotor reflexes and the right one —

---

[1] The contemporary science hasn't find yet the foreseen by ancient yogis interlacements of Ida and Pingala. Maybe such inventions are still to come.

for venous ones. Both trunks segmentally form more or less important plexus (corresponding to chakras — A. S.), local control centres, all connected to the single subdominant system. From bottom-up these plexus are: 1) plexus pudendus or pi. sacralis, responsible for visceral, mostly vascular plexus of cavernous bodies and the inferior part of the rectum; 2) plexus lumbalis responsible for vegetative reflexes of urogenital system and legs; 3) solar plexus — a huge plexus of nerve tissue, located in the front part of the abdominal aorta in the form of complicated mass of nerve ganglia and fibres, partly filling the Halleri tripes, formed by three major arteries of abdominal cavity, coming out from abdominal aorta: liver, spleen and stomach arteries. They form the lowest part of the plexus in the abdomen.

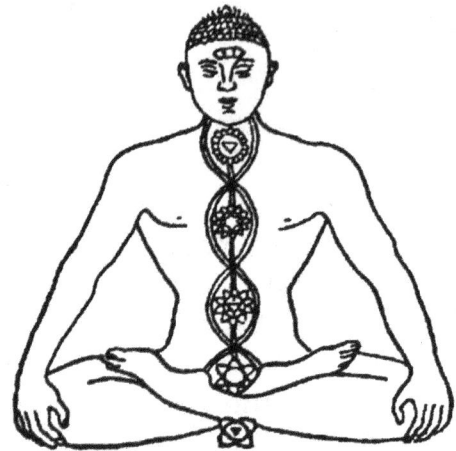

PICTURE 4. Ida and Pingala
Wrong image of Ida and Pingala, given in the majority of Western textbooks on yoga. (This figure was borrowed from book by S. Esudian, E. Haich «Yoga for modern human health»).
In fact, Ida and Pingala start on the petals of the third eye and do not cross at muladhara

Going up, there is a heart-portal plexus: a centre of primary importance, one of the major apparatus, controlling overall blood circulation, except for the circulation in the cerebrum, with which the aortic plexus is associated. This plexus is boarded by a stellar cervical. It is one of the inner apparatus, controlling blood circulation in cerebrum.

At the level of larynx (Adam's apple) there is a plexus of carotid and its famous carotid body — one of the important regulators of cerebrum blood circulation. On the skull base there is an anatomically unseen, but physiologically important plexus of craniocerebral nerves having vegetative innervations, above all vagus nerve and trigeminus (the 10th and the 5th pairs).

Above all — there is the brain with its mosaic cortex, like a flower with many petals of different parts and structures.

The activity period of each channel counts 60–90 minutes, the basic biological human's rhythm. The change in activity, as already said above, can be traced by the change of the «active» nostril. Longer or shorter periods indicate an illness. The same rhythm is well known to a contemporary medicine, as a sleep cycle. After a half of a cycle the active nostril and the channel change. At this moment for some minutes switches in the central energy channel, Sushumna, going long the backbone. In this rare moment we are completely balanced. Then the balance shifts again.

28

«Svaradoya shastra» gives some detailed recommendations regarding favourable and non-favourable activities at the time of each nostril (when the right nostril is open one should perform some eager activity, when the left one — to rest, to think about eternal things etc.), analyses how malfunctions of a natural cycle relate to illnesses, gives some techniques of compulsory changes of nostril.

Hindus think that you can use a cotton tampon to change the active nostril, if needed. Imagine, a person is tired, but has to go on. He puts a cotton tampon into his left nostril, the right nostril opens and his reserves are released. Hindu were very pragmatic. A woman likes more a man when she has the left nostril active and he — the right one. It was also thought that conceiving of a boy or a girl also depends on the open nostril. If in the right moment man had a right nostril open and a woman a left one, they conceive a boy. If vice versa — a girl.

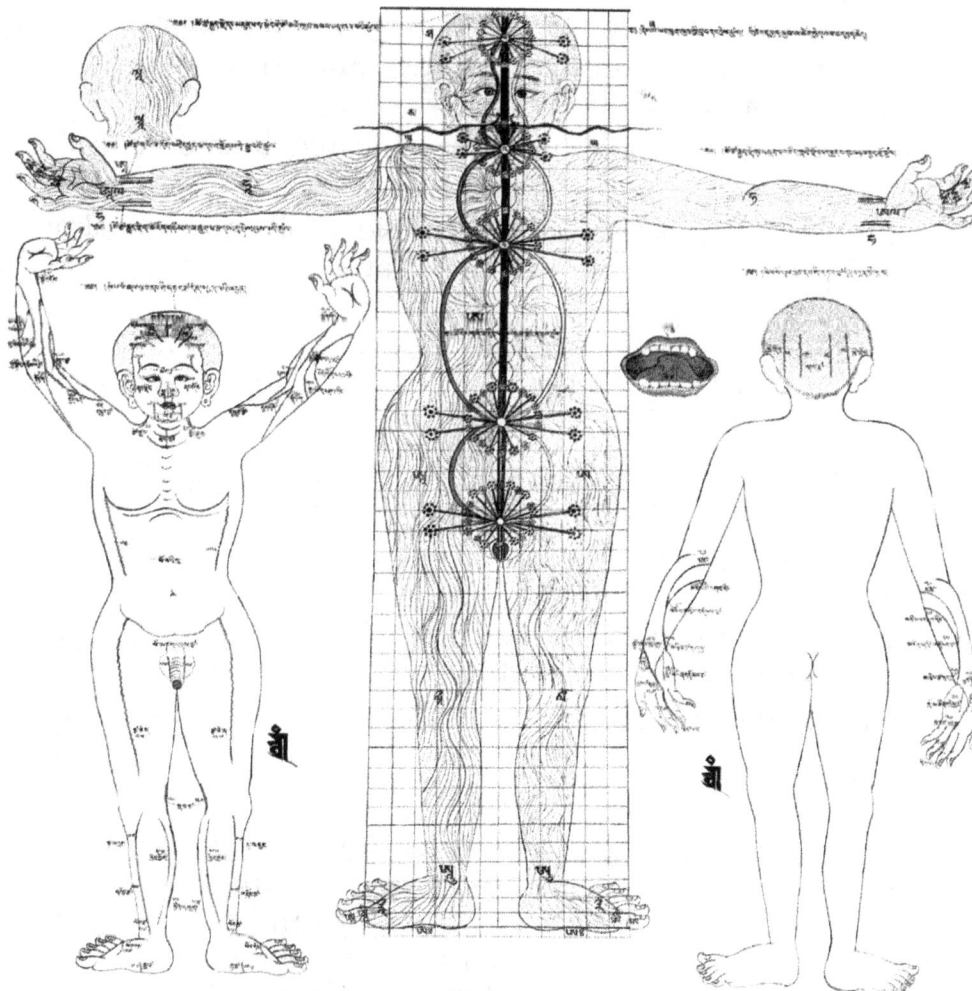

PICTURE 5. Ida and Pingala
Picture from the «Atlas of Tibetan Medicine»

Other energy channels

In addition to all above said ancient treatises were defining a lot of minor energy channels (Sanskrit: *nadi*). Thus «Shiva svarodaya» says:

32. From the navel 72 000 nadis emanate and go through the whole body...

36. From all the nadi 10 are the most known. Among them *Ida, Pingala* and *Sushumna* are the most important.

37. The rest are: *Gandkhari, Puusha, Yashashvini, Alambusha, Kukhuu* and the tenth — *Shankhini*.

38. Ida nadi — the left side of the body, pingala — the right side, sushumna in the centre, and Gandkhari — the left eye.

39. Hastijihva — the right eye, Puusha — the right ear, Yashsshvini — in the left ear, Alambusha — the face.

40. Kukhuu — reproductive organs, Shankhini — anal. This is how 10 nadi are located in a body.

41. Ida, Pingala and Sushumna are located in the central part of the body.

42. I told you the names of nadis. Now I'll tell you about vaya (types of air), related to nadi. These are Prana, Apana, Samana, Udana, Viana.

43. And *Naga, Kurma, Krikara, Devadatta, Dhananiaia* — additional pranas. Prana is located in the heart, while apana vaya — in emunctories.

44. Samana is located in navel. Udana — in larynx. Viana fills all the body. 10 vayu are also very important.

45. I told you about five major vayu. Now I'll tell you about the rest five vayu and their location.

46. Naga vayu controls the belching; Kurma — the winking, Krikara — the sneezing, Devadatta — the yawning.

47. Dhananiaia fills all after the death. While a person is alive these 10 vaya operate in all nadi.

From this extract we can conclude that the described channels mostly sure relate with the nerve fibres going from the brain and medulla, responsible for reflex arches and controlling breathing, winking, secretion and other partly voluntary processes. Apparently these channels have physical, etheric and astral manifestation. The existence of the last one becomes understandable, if we recall that a need to do each of these activities (as winking for example) is perceived as a **wish.**

Energy channels in Chinese tradition

Chinese tradition (as well *as acupuncture therapy*) uses a slightly different system of energy channels. This tradition defines anterior and posterior centre meridians (the most important), 12 major meridians, related with organs, and 28 lo-channels, connecting the above mentioned[1].

Energy (*qi* in Chinese tradition) circulates in the said 12 meridians during the day, forming a circadian biological rhythm. Medicine many times tried to make a connection between Chinese meridians and organic structures, but the complete correlation has never been found. However acupuncture is «working». Moreover the presence of points and channels can be felt by extrasensory methods. Probably the Chinese system of meridians is located on the etheric level.

Some acupuncture channels are activated while doing yoga exercises (see chapter «Yoga-therapy. Some principles of building a yoga complex»).

---

[1]   More details you can find in any book on acupuncture. Schemes of muscle-tendon meridians, a physical analogue of acupuncture ones are given in the appendix 1.

TYPES OF YOGA EXERCISES AND THEIR MECHANISMS OF INFLUENCE

In yoga there are following types of exercises: **asanas, pranayamas, bandhas, mudras, kriyas, mantras** and **meditation techniques.**

Asanas

Patanjali defines asana as a «comfortable and pleasant posture». Some modern practitioners might think, this definition is a mocking. Indeed some yoga positions demand considerable agility, force, stretching and can hardly be called «comfortable and pleasant». Such a paradox can be probably explained by the fact that at a time of Patanjali yogins were practicing an insignificant number of asanas, with no difficult ones, that are given today by modern schools. In «Hatha Yoga pradipika» there is a list of 11 asanas for body strengthening and 4 meditative ones. In the first group there are: Svastikasana, Gomughasana, Virasana, Kurmasana, Kukutasana, Uttana Kurmasana, Dhanurasana, Matiasana, Pashimotta-nasana, Maiurasana, Shavasana. In the second one: Siddhasana, Padmasana, Simhasana, Bhadrasana. Such a limited number of exercises wasn't explained by the low development of the system, but by the clear understanding that yoga isn't a technique for hypertrophied body development. **Asanas are not the ultimate goal, but an intermediate instrument that yoga offers a person for his spiritual evolution.** In my opinion, to practice yoga efficiently, aiming for both physical health and inner work, some 10 asanas are enough, although their list will vary for different people, depending on their physical and psychological features.

«Gheranda samhita» gives 32 asanas, which are still considered as the most important and frequently used:

1. Siddhasana (siddha pose)
2. Padmasana (lotus pose)
3. Bhadrasana (easy pose)
4. Muktasana (liberation pose)

5. Vajrasana (diamond pose)
6. Svastikasana (Svastika pose)
7. Simhasana (Lion pose)
8. Gomukhasana (cow head pose)
9. Virasana (hero pose)
10. Dhanurasana (bow pose)
11. Shavasana (corpse pose)
12. Guptasana (secret pose)
13. Matsiasana (fish pose)
14. Matsiendrasana (Matsiendra pose)
15. Gorakshasana (Gorokshi pose)
16. Pashimottanasana (forward inclination pose) bending
17. Utkatasana (squatting pose)
18. Sankatasana (hard pose)
19. Maiurasana (peacock pose)
20. Kakkutasana (cock pose)
21. Kurmasana (turtle pose)
22. Uttanakurmasana (standing turtle pose)
23. Vrikshasana (tree pose)
24. Mandukasana (frog pose)
25. Uttanamandukasana (standing frog pose)
26. Garudasana (eagle pose)
27. Vrisabhasana (bull pose)
28. Shalabhasana (grasshopper pose)
29. Makarasana (Makara pose)
30. Ushtrasana (camel pose)
31. Bhujangasana (cobra pose)
32. Yogasana (yogin pose)

As some yoga exercises are difficult to classify (for example, why yoga-mudra is considered as mudra while it looks like asana), let's try to give asana a more exact definition, basing on significant specific criteria.

Asana is an exercise, helping to control energy and physiological processes in our body through redistribution of stretching, squeezing and tension in our body. Asana can have a specific sequence of entering and exiting it, but it is obligatory to stay in it statically for some time.

Asana influences mostly **our physical and etheric body,** hardly touching our emotional sphere.

How asanas influence on our body

Mechanical influence of asanas

Most of asanas activate many muscles, in particular those that are hardly used in our everyday life. This explains special complication of asanas. Unlike other exercises they aimed at **local** influence on various parts of our body. Doing common physical exercises we chaotically involve our main muscles. How can we activate a strictly defined group of muscles? By taking a special position. The more complicated asanas are, the more precisely they influence on local groups of muscles. This way we can save our energy, otherwise wasted for «unneeded» muscles.

Humoral mechanism

From the physical point of view the human body can be presented as an interrelated system of cavities, filled with liquids and gases. Yoga exercises significantly and very selectively influence on the volume of these cavities, and as a result, the pressure in them. So these exercises provide a particular inside massage of our viscera. Understanding of the hydraulic aspect of asanas gives us hints on how to do them: as each asana changes intracavitary pressure, while liquid's mobility is limited anatomically, so **the speed of entering asana and exiting it must be enough to let intracavitary pressure stabilise, i.e. we must enter and exit a pose slowly and stay in it long enough.** If this condition is not respected, asanas become at the best the ordinary fitness for muscles.

Another humoral mechanism of influence is a **change of hydrostatic pressure.** As we know, the formula of hydrostatic pressure is:

$$P = pgh,$$

where p is liquid density, g — acceleration of gravity, h — height of a liquid column.

That is why most of asanas change hydrostatic pressure on certain organs. Especially it is true for inverted poses like *Sirshasana, sarvangasana* and *halasana.* This mechanism of influence was studied by D. Ebert [p.].

To reinforce this effect some poses are accompanied with udiana bandha, which raises the corporal pressure simply by reducing the torso's volume.

There is another aspect of humoral mechanism that should be mentioned. Citing another extract from the book of the famous yoga researcher D. Ebert: «The growing intravascular pressure, produced by raising intra-abdominal pressure shift s the liquids exchange balance to the intensification of filtration. As a result: the clotting of blood, the hypostasis in interstition and reinforcement of lymphatic outflow. Mukerji and Spiegelhoff [1971] describe a slight growth of red cells and leucocytes in blood after performing udiana-bandha and pavana-muktasana. These results can be interpreted as a result of blood clotting due to the growing share of filtration in tissues». From all above said we can conclude that drinking a lot of water, suggested in yoga system, is an absolute must for a regular practitioner. Moreover, **practice of hatha yoga is inseparable from the system of cleansing procedures.**

Psychosomatic mechanism

Since ancient times people knew that human body and soul are interrelated. First attempts to diagnose person's character by his outward appearance were done long time ago: for instance physiognomies — the art of telling person's character and fate by his face; chiromancy — by the lines on his palm; phrenology — by the particularities of his skull etc, but the contemporary psychology brought up this question quite recently. Only in the late 1900s W. Reich, W. James, A. Lowen together with other famous psychotherapists found out that human psyche is projected on our physical body in a form of constitutional type, muscle contractions. The contrary is also true: certain work with the body can change human's psychological state. According to contemporary knowledge, the projective connection, correlating human psyche and body looks like this:

Neck and throat are related with intellect, the ability to speak out your thoughts, with the right to have your own opinion, take independent decisions. Contractions in the throat zone are often related with the fact that a person «suppresses» his wish to express his offence or other overwhelming emotions. This can cause thyroid dysfunctions. Contractions in the back of the neck, neck osteochondrosis show an excessive yoke of responsibility taken by a person and sometimes by his wish «to hide», to draw his head in, to become invisible.

Chest and heart are related with the sensual sphere. Contractions in this area are related with the inability to show freely and sincerely such feelings as love, dislike, sympathy etc. The most common type of contraction in this zone is the inability to breathe with full lungs, i.e. with the even widening of thorax at all sides and with rising collar-bones with the straight spine. Typical diseases arising as a result of such emotional problems are heart attacks, osteochondrosis. The inability to rejoice all life manifestations causes lung diseases; offences unexpressed for a long time cause asthma.

Stomach zone relates with the need to dominate, with power, recognition, aggression. If these needs are frustrated, a person has weak abdominal muscles, flabby belly, sometimes diseases of abdominal organs. Tension in lower back muscles relates with the fear of attack.

Pelvis zone relates with the need of sex and pleasures. People with rigid pelvis usually don't allow themselves to have pleasures. Bad stretching of legs has also to do with this problem. Typical disorders in this case are lower back osteochondrosis, bladder and genitals diseases. Greed, craving to save at one's own expense cause constipations and haemorrhoids.

Face except for the will centre on the forehead reflects projections of all other zones. So the head is projected on the forehead, the throat on the nose, the heart on the upper lip, the stomach on the teeth, the pelvis on the lower lip, cheeks — are arms, elbows are on tumours. Rigidity of consequent zones of the face shows the presence of contractions in the respective zones of the body with following psychological problems.

It's easy to notice **that the given projection network reminds us human chakral system** — basic energy model, used in yoga; while muscle contractions and other abnormalities are physical expressions of energy defects of chakras. From this point of view the main task of physical yoga exercises, in particular asanas, is obvious: **by influencing physical body to change human's psychological state, to restore his energetic integrity and to develop his chakral system.**

Psychosomatic influence of asanas uses another mechanism — **breaking** *pathogenic arches*. Most of people during their life «collect» non-adaptive motor stereotypes: for example, by clutching your fist you'll notice clenching your teeth. Practicing asanas we can break these stereotypes, significantly raising our motor and psychological liberty, also making it possible to save a lot of energy (see chapter «Psychological work in asanas»).

Reflex mechanism

There are some reflex mechanisms that provide additional influence of asanas. The easiest of them is changes in local homodynamic — the compensatory intensification in blood circulation after stretching and pressing. Derma-visceral and motor-visceral reflexes, influencing directly functions of different organs, are more complicated. They exist because sensitive nerves of viscera, skin regions (Zakharin-Ged zones) and muscles interlace on the level of medulla segments, corresponding chakras. As a result the tension in certain muscles and stimulation of certain zones of skin influence organs.

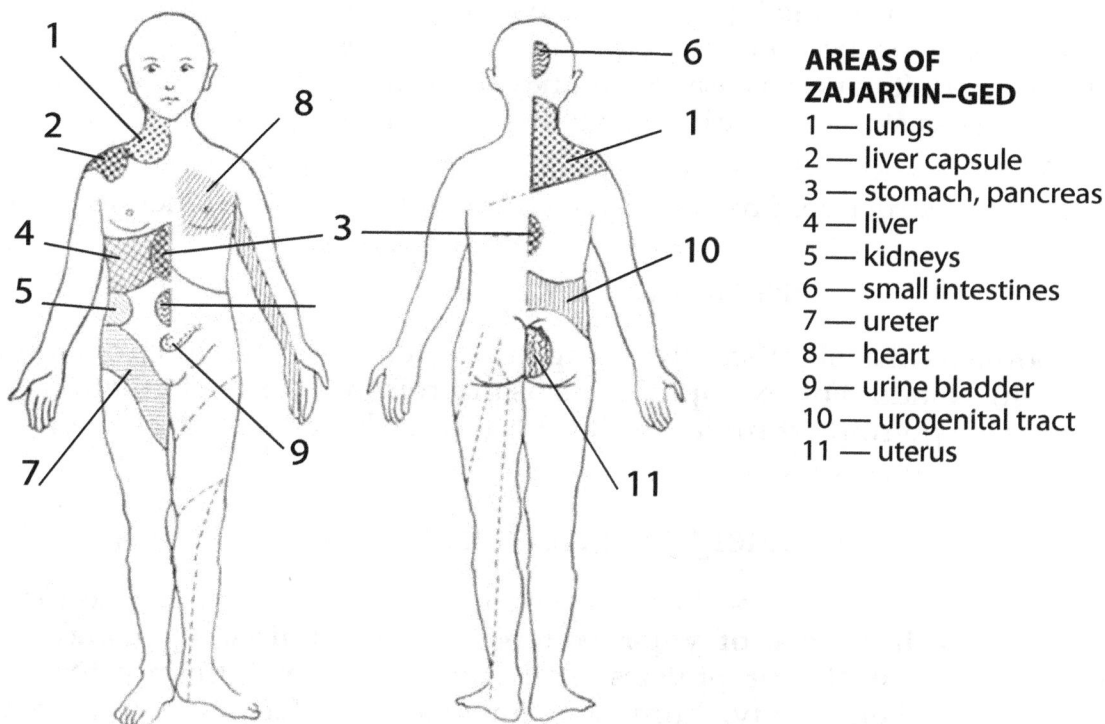

AREAS OF ZAJARYIN–GED
1 — lungs
2 — liver capsule
3 — stomach, pancreas
4 — liver
5 — kidneys
6 — small intestines
7 — ureter
8 — heart
9 — urine bladder
10 — urogenital tract
11 — uterus

Stress mechanism

Anyone who practiced asanas, could notice that unlike Patanjali said, most of them are unnatural postures, i.e. unusual for everyday life. Actually asanas expressly put our body in a brand new, unusual posture, causing microstress. Such stress positively influences on our body stimulating our limbic system, certainly, if microstress does not grow into a macro[1] one. From this mechanism we can conclude some practical rules:

1. Asana will «work», if you make an extra effort, i.e. make it an unusual position. This extra effort can be caused by an express stretching (but, of course, without pain), by staying in a pose for slightly longer time, than our body's reflex wants, or by optionally changing the natural rhythm of breathing etc.

---

[1] L. Kh. Garkavi in 1979, developing the teaching on stress, found out that in response to the action of weak irritants (low doses), regardless of their quality, physiological adaptation reaction develops — the reaction of training; to the action of irritants of medium force (dose) — activation reaction; to the action of strong irritant — stress. The reaction of training and the reaction of activation represent those adaptive reactions, which are met during normal body life. These reactions are non-specific basis for physiological processes, as well as to the stress — non-specific various pathological processes.

2. Our body quickly adapts to usual stresses, that's why exercises of the same type become less efficient. Complexes should be reviewed and perfected. It concerns asanas, pranayamas, as well as the rest of techniques such as stressful purifying methods like fasting, and meditations.

3. Too stressful performance gives the opposite result. Macrostresses are destructive. That is why we must always know when to stop.

Hormonal mechanism

Some asanas significantly change the intensity of blood circulation in certain glands. For example, matsiasana reinforces the circulation in the zone of thyroid, stimulating its work and, by activated hormones, influencing the entire body.

Energetic mechanism

All the described mechanisms certainly work not only for asanas. However the **influence of yoga exercises is not limited by usual fitness, by work with our physics.** The main object of influence for asanas is our etheric body, human's vital energy. Many contemporary occult-extrasensory schools speak about working with energy and try to master it by consciousness practising of visualisation. Some people succeed.. but in most cases they got caught in their own fantasy. Actually it is not difficult to tell the difference between an illusionary etheric work and a realistic one. Etheric energy intensively influences on physical body — when the energy is moving, it has some concrete somatic appearances: in activated zones body temperature changes, appears inner vibration (when there is too much energy in a zone), pain disappear. If these effects are not present, you don't really work with energy.

> 2.12. In the beginning there is perspiration, in the middle stage there is quivering, and in the last or third stage, one obtains steadiness; and then the breath should be made steady or motionless.
>
> *Hatha Yoga Pradipika*

It's quite possible to work with energy by your will, but it is a level, which takes a long time to reach. However in yoga there is another common way to master energy, using correlation between our physical and etheric bodies. A correctly done posture arouses some energy movement in the ether.

Here are some principles, describing the interrelation of our physical and etheric bodies.

1. The energy moves from the pressed zones to the stretched one, from the relaxed to the tensed one.

2. Energy moves by the channels. A channel is a stretched line on our body. A healthy person has natural channels called muscle-tendon

38

meridians (see Appendix 1.), but, if we have energetic blocks, the energy can pass out of these channels.

3. A channel is open only if all its parts are open, i.e. If it is equally stretched at all its length. If it is closed in any place, it is completely closed, like water cannot run in a hose, if it is stepped on in one single place.

4. Any energy movement in a channel **is always** accompanied with physical effects long all the channel. Most often it is a feeling of warmth or even heat moving up your body[1]. If a channel is blocked there can be an effect of «pricking», as when blood comes back to a dumb limb. When a block is passed the pricking is changed into heat.

So there are the following energy mechanisms of asanas influence:

1. Opening and «purification» of channels. They are usually blocked by a certain quantity of «frozen» etheric energy long the channel. Such «chunks» of energy usually relate to some blocked emotions, i.e. astral energy, around which the ether energy crystallizes and makes a block. On a physical level such blocks are seen as chronic muscle contractions, tensions and pressures. Actually the work with these blocks can start from the astral body (by catharsis reacting of restrained emotions), as well as through our etheric and physical bodies, i.e. with the help of asanas. No doubt the most efficient is cooperation of all methods, which will be discussed in chapter «Psychological work in asanas».

2. Energy repartition of ether from the parts where it is excessive to those zones that lack it. In particular, «patching up» of holes in ether, stimulation of oppressed chakras and sadatation of excited ones.

3. «Working out», i.e. **energizing of problem zones.** A low energy in a zone can be explained by body's constitutional type or by a set-up received while growing-up and is expressed by an obvious weakness of a part. For example, a «swan neck», thin arms and legs etc. In a lighter manifestation a weaker part (mostly a limb) has more tendency to freeze. Practicing asanas, these parts can become more energetic.

4. General energy circulation intensification. Most of esoteric traditions think that personal strength and energy level of a person depends not on how much energy he has in subtle bodies, but on the intensification of its flow in his body. Qigong masters say that a common human has string-width energy channels, while a qigong master can have them as wide as the finger. The speed at which energy moves changes too. It can be easily proved by the following observation. Practicing yoga correctly, a yogin has to spend in a pose less and less time to get the same physiological effect. So, if a newcomer has the heat move up his spine in a one minute and a half after exiting Bhujangasana, in a year of practice you need just 10–15 seconds.

---

[1]   I suppose it is this heat that Indians used to call «tapas».

Types of asanas

Depending on a mechanism of influence there are six types of asanas:

- stretching;
- pivoting;
- strengthening;
- inverted;
- pressing;
- equilibration.

Stretching asanas influence our meridians, located on the forward and backward part of the body. Among forward stretchings are: *Bhujangasana, Ushtrasana, Chakrasana.* Backward stretchings are: *Yoga Mudra, Pashimottanasana, Padakhastasana.*

Pivoting asanas work with diagonal meridians. Among them: *Arthamatsiendrasana, Trikonasana, Parivritta Trikonasana* and *Parivritta parsvakonasana.*

Strengthening asanas don't stretch channel, but condense the ether by natural movement of energy to the strained zone. Among them are: *Purvotanasana, Salabkh-* and *Arthasalabhasana, Firabhadrasana, Utkatasana, Viparita karani, Kukutasana, Artha navasana* and *Paripura navasana.*

Inverted asanas change energy and liquids circulation in the body under the influence of gravity. These are: *Sirshasana, Sarpasana, Halasana, Karnapidasasana.*

Pressing and squeezing out asanas squeeze energy out of some zones by physical pressure on it. These are *Gomukhasana, Maiurasana.*

Equilibration asanas influence our body by activating certain muscles, baroceptors related to them, brain and limbic system — to keep balance.

Actually there are much more asanas. Moreover each asana has its countless modifications. You can also make combined asanas, having characters of each type, but the aim of this book is not to give the complete list of asanas. Dogmatism is fatal for a spiritual teaching. We'll try to look down the origins and to understand principles, underlying hatha yoga; using them practitioner will know, how to construct asanas and other exercises according to his own task and his personal psychophysiological and energetic features.

It's interesting to note that in asanas, described in «Hatha Yoga Pradipika», there are 1–2 exercises of each type.

Pranayamas[1]

Human breath is a process controlled by both the brain and the consciousness. Breath is a «bridge» between our biological and spiritual nature. The way we breathe, our particularities, depth, the muscles we use, directly relate with our consciousness. No wonder we use such sayings as «with bated breath», «take one's breath away», «a lump in the throat» etc. If **our consciousness is still** (or even the psyche in general, because subconsciousness also influences it) **our breath is stable, deep with even rhythm.** On the contrary, as soon as our physical state or the direction of consciousness flow changes, rhythm and type of breath changes too. At a limit there is a breath breakdown, a temporary breath-holding, not controlled by our consciousness. For example, if we try to lift something heavy, we have a breakdown in a form of tension and groaning, but sometimes such a breakdown occurs when the object to lift isn't heavy at all. It is the attitude: the object is too heavy in person's mind. This is an example of mind breakdown. The same breakdown would lead to the similar breath breakdown that can happen, if we think about a physiologically difficult situation.

A person can think that he is absolutely calm, but any exterior observer can easily see, if it's true, by the way he breathes. Our breathing shows our real emotional state. And vice versa by controlling our breath, we can learn to control our emotional state. The detailed knowledge about chakral system and principles of psychosomatic interrelation can help us to minutely analyse the current state of any person's psyche, just by observing and listening to his breath.

But for goals of yoga it is also important to know, that the counter principle works too: **consciously controlling and keeping certain breathing rhythm, we form a defined in advance state of awareness.** This is the principle underlying the next type of yoga exercises — **pranayamas. Pranayama is a breath control.** «Yoga kundalia-upanishada» says «there are two reasons making our mind wander — *vasanas* (desires, caused by secretly impressed feelings) and *the breath. If* our desires can be mastered, the other can be controlled. From these two the first to master must be our breath».

So **pranayamas** are breathing exercises. «Hatha Yoga Pradipika» describes 8 pranayamas: *Suria Bheda, Udjai, Sitcari, Sitali, Bhastrica, Bhramari, Murchha and Plavini*. Sometimes in ancient yoga pranayama meant a breath-hold. Modern yoga counts dozens of pranayamas and their variations, such as: full breath, quick pranayamas, slow, dynamic pranayamas. On our physical body pranayama makes less impact, than asanas. **It mainly aims at etheric and astral bodies,** i.e. vitality and emotional sphere.

---

[1]   Curiously like in English «prana» means both «air» and some life force, vital energy.

Influence mechanism of breath exercises, pranayamas in particular, is based on the following principles.

1. The changing of ratio of oxygen and carbonic acid in our body. Raising concentration of oxygen, we activate inhibitory processes by intensive breathing and lung hyperventilation. The rising concentration of carbonic acid is achieved by holding our breath, and in different phases results in activating certain zones of our brain. For instance, by raising the level of CO_2 by pranayamas, we activate all hypercapnic chemoreceptors and our respiratory centre, arises the reciprocal intensification of ventilation, that is why the successfulness of the respiratory training is defined by the eventual slow rising of *hypercapnia*. Only in this case we can achieve a growth in chemoreceptors and neurons of respiratory centre resistance to a hypercapnic stimulation, fortifying respiratory system in physical load and in closed spaces (transport etc.). In the long run hypercapnia adaptation also raises compensatory capacities of buffer systems, favours removal of hyperventilate disorders, hypercapnia, normalisation of carbonic acid in tissues and cell metabolism optimisation.

These effects were researched by modern physicians, who came to same conclusions, as those acknowledged in ancient yoga. The foresaid Garkavi and his co-authors showed that hypercapnia can be used as a factor of raising a non-specific resistance of the body. Another researcher Pavlenko wrote that hypercapnia normally has pathogenic effect, but till a certain moment activates the respiratory centre, playing its sanogeneric role.

The same research was conducted in the «opposite» branch — excessive oxygen. Thus researches of brain activity in the state of *holotropic breathwork,* conducted in the Institute of high nerve activity have showed that during such breathing there is an activation of the back left and forward right parts of the brain, the so-called «axis of superconscious». The same are activated in the state of creativity. In the normal state lobe zones of the left hemisphere and back of the right one are activated (cognitive axis).

Combining the lasting ratio of inhalation-hold-exhalation-hold, we can reach a strictly defined ratio of oxygen/carbonic acid content in our blood, thus getting into various «calibrated» states. Such method becomes even more efficient by a direct rhythmic influence on the brain by nerve endings, located in nasopharynx. Methods of rhythmical breathwork were used not only in yoga, but also in magical practices, qigong, martial arts and shaman practices.

2. Enabling different groups of muscles in breathing. The interrelation between various human muscles, in particular, respiratory muscles, was noticed and introduced in contemporary theory of psychosomatics by A. Lowen, although it is evident from the structure of chakral system. The main point of such correlation is that **while breathing, people don't use muscles, located at the level of their disrupted or weak chakras. The opposite is also true; if while breathing we «switch on» certain muscles, we activate the chakra itself.** The additional effect can be produced by straining (working out) of different groups of respiratory muscles.

3. **Reflex effect on the brain by influencing on olfactory and other receptors,** located in respiratory tracts. Some researches think that *limbic system* on the one hand relates with our emotional sphere, on the other — with the organs»[1] work control, in its evolutionary base has a rhinencephalon. That is why the air, rhythmically passing through the nose, puts the limbic system in a particular state, which tells upon the general state of the body — physical and emotional. Author does not possess more detailed information about deeper neurophysic researches, that is why, choosing cycles, we should trust our empirical observation and reflection — just like ancient yogins.

4. **Hydraulic brain and viscera massage.** Pranayamas, especially those done intensively (like kalabhati and Bhastrika) create certain changes in pressure — in the body and in the head, causing the effect of their inner massage. From this principle we can conclude that **there is a minimum speed of doing these pranayamas, at which they cause a needed effect.**

5. **Reflex impact over sympathetic and parasympathetic nervous system.** In classical yoga it is believed that breathing through the right nostril is stimulating and favours dissociation processes in our body (Sun breathing). Breathing through the left nostril is soothing and favours assimilation processes (Moon breathing). That is why, the express activating of a nostril or the specific order of changing nostrils is an important element in yoga, practically its «visiting card».

> 2.7. Sitting in the Padmâsana posture the Yogi should fill in the air through the left nostril (closing the right one); and, keeping it confined according to one's ability, it should be expelled slowly through the surya (right nostril).
>
> 2.8. Then, drawing in the air through the surya slowly, the belly should be filled, and after performing Kumbhaka as before, it should be expelled slowly through the chandra (left nostril).
>
> *Hatha Yoga Pradipika*

6. **Effect of psychosomatic correspondence on the inner respiratory system.** The basic system of psychosomatic correspondence described above is not the only one. Other local systems related to chakras

---

[1] Probably this interlacement of functions is a physical basis of psychosomatic correlation existence.

can also be found. For example, seven cervical vertebras are projected to seven chakras. The same correlation exists in the respiratory system: more outlying zones of nasopharynx are related with inferior chakras, and deeper ones — with the upper chakras. Upper zones are related with the brain, lower zones — with the body. Combining aerodynamic types of breathing (for example, by a certain pose of the head or the tension in nostrils), we can influence any particular zone. Another way to use this mechanism is concentration on different feelings in the nose, i.e. activating different receptors, and therefore different parts of the brain.

Breathing can be successfully combined with meditation. There is a number of meditation techniques, based on consciousness structuring — not always on relaxation, — with the help of breathing. The most simple is the one, when a practitioner sits down and starts listening to his breathing. In one of the Shastras this technique is described as: «Listening to your breath, you listen to the breath of the Universe». One should sit and breathe — nothing more. This meditation quickly helps to come into a state of trace.

Bandhas

«*Bandha*» is a Sanskrit word for a «lock», which characterises the meaning and mechanism of its influence. **Bandhas block certain energy flows and liquids transference related to them,** that is why most often bandhas are done in those exercises that change corporal pressure. In classic yoga there are three main bandhas: *Jalandhara Bandha, Uddiyana Bandha and Mula Bandha*[1].

Jalandhara Bandha closes the energy inflow to the head and prevents from high intracranial pressure in exercises, raising corporal pressure — such as Kumbhaka. Indeed, try to «unlock» Jalandhara Bandha and you'll feel a hydraulic hit in your head, i.e. a sudden change in your intracranial pressure, resulting in «birds» before your eyes or some noise in your head.

Uddiyana Bandha condenses energy in Manipura and directs it to Anahata. That is why after Bhastrikas we do kumbhaka and uddiyana bandha. All excessive energy, pumped by Bhastrikas to Manipura, is transferred to Anahata.

Moreover uddiyana bandha positively influences the organs of abdominal cavity owing to mechanic massage.

Mula Bandha condenses energy in lower chakras. It is also done whenever there is an excessive pressure or a concentration of energy, to stop energy from flowing into earth. Moreover mula bandha prevents

---

[1]   Although Maja Bandha is also called «bandha», it has a different essence.

the outflow of the energy from Muladhara (related to vital force) to other people. If at a contact with someone your limbs start freezing, you're chilling and physically (not emotionally) feeling worse, probably there is such an outflow, and mula bandha can help to cease these symptoms.

Mechanically mula bandha stimulates internal genitalia, favours intimate muscles development, helping men to control ejaculation and women — to make the orgasm more intensive and to massage penis during coitus.

Kriya

«*Kriya*» is a Sanskrit word for «action», that is why lately it is used for many dynamic yoga practices, but in reality kriya is an exercise, that makes a dynamic impact, actually, **a viscera massage.** Kriya is a «know-how» of yoga — in other systems of physical culture there's nothing of this kind. Among kriya techniques are: *Uddiana Bandha Kriya, Nauli Kriya*. Kriyas are also cleansing techniques, which have to do with niyama. They are aimed to clean our body from harmful substances. A special attention is drawn to cleansing of digestive tract, blood and other systems. There are six types of cleansings: *Netî, Dhautî, Naulî, Basti, Kapâlabhâtî, Trâtaka*. Every type has its procedures and cleansing techniques. Principles of action of these exercises are in most cases obvious.

Mudras

Mudras are usually understood as a certain gesture. This understanding is formed under the influence of Buddhist tradition, where hand gestures were widely used. But strictly speaking, in classic yoga the term «*mudra*» is much wider: it can be performed with entire body, like the already mentioned *yoga mudra, shaktichelani mudra* and others, although they are more rare. Mudras can be performed by the eyes (like in *sambhavi mudra, vaishnavi mudra*), by the tongue (*nabho mudra, khechari mudra*) and even by the anus (*ashvini mudra*)[1]. **Mudras are mostly practiced in meditation techniques** and are rarely involved in physical exercise. This is understandable, because **mudras make a** very **subtle effect** on people, **on their emotional plane** (astral body). Their mechanism of influence also has to do with psychosomatic correlation. To understand this mechanism let's look at mudras' closest relative — gestures. Good old gestures constitute an important part of communication. **Gestures are directly related to the current emo-**

---

[1] Gherenda samhita enlists 25 mudras, but, if to count those from other origins, they are a lot more.

tional state and perform an energy movement in the aura. Mudras use the opposite principle, intensifying movement of a needed energy, forming a needed state. Look, what are hand positions of people sitting in public transport. Sometimes their hands are interlaced in complicated exotic mudras, but not due to high popularity of exsoterism. This is one of the natural forms of body's autoregulation, noticed and made to serve by ancient practitioners. The mudra's capacity to activate emotions was used in classical Indian theatre and dancing art, where mudras were called «hasts».

In some «popular» sources about yoga you can find the belief that mudras influence the body by «enclosing our channels». By channels they mean meridians by Chinese medicine (acupuncture). Indeed, four of these channels end in our hands, but what good to enclose a channel of lungs with a channel of small intestine like in djanana mudra? I don't know any cases, when mudras strongly influenced the physical body, vegetative system, i.e. etheric body, that is why I believe such an explanation is far-fetched.

Mudras have a very subtle influence on the body. If you compare our organism with a refurbishment in a house, mudras are the thin emery-paper, which you use after having worked with a plane, sandpapered and varnished, and now you get it polished, but, if you took a thin emery-paper when you still have splinters everywhere, the effect from it would be insignificant. **Mudras are exercises of the advanced level.**

By types there are enclosing mudras, blocking energy outflow from chakra; dhiana mudras, helping to keep a certain state in various meditations; and **excretive,** concentrating astral energy outside of the body.

Vibration techniques (Mantras)

One of the most ancient techniques in human's history is repeating of mantras — certain sound combinations, resonance with particular parts of our brain and body. According to modern studies of neuropsychologists, practice of mudras really changes relative amplitudes of brain rhythms, providing altered states of consciousness. They should not be confused with prayers and other forms of autosuggestion, because they can have no meaning (although some of them do have it). Some mantras have a symbolic meaning, for example, six syllables of Tibetan mantra *Om mani padme hum* correspond to six worlds of Buddhist cosmogony, but it is an exception.

Unfortunately mechanisms of mantra influence are not sufficiently studied. Maybe a key to understanding are researches of phonosemantics as for primary meanings of sounds, as well as the scheme of how different parts of the body correspond to different sounds.

There is another mechanism of mantra influence — resonance effect on endocrine and nervous vegetative systems. Indeed, singing various sounds, we can form our standing to have the maximum vibration amplitude over the needed zones. Thus mantras can perform an inner massage to our endocrine glands (see «Advanced pranayamas»).

Note that human's history has other analogues of reading mantras. Hence a well-known musical instrument of Northern people — Jew's-harp, uses the skull as the resonator, which makes it possible to localize acoustic vibrations of maximum amplitude in certain parts of brain, stimulating their activity.

In Indian tradition there were four ways (or stages) of reading mantras:

First stage — singing mantra aloud distinctly;

Second stage — mantra is whispered with distinct articulation;

Third stage — mantra is read mentally;

Fourth stage — the highest — lines of mantra are not pronounced, but a practitioner takes the respective state.

There are also some less known ways to use mantras. One of them is a brusque shouting out of certain sounds. For instance, in Tibetan yoga to relieve depression, they were shouting out mantra «phat». In Japan there were mantras «os» and «kiay». These practices demand an articulate pronunciation and correlating mantras with breathing.

Another technique that can be considered as mantra is listening to inhaling and exhaling of the air. In Indian tradition it is believed that when you inhale the air, it makes the sound «so» or «sah», and when you exhale — the sound «ham».

Meditative practices in Yoga

Psychological aspect

Methods of meditations aim at mastering psyche functions by concentrating attention (passive meditation) or will (active meditation). Not only methods, but the ways to meditate are so different, not to mention that by «meditation» we often understand absolutely different processes, so let's try to define a typology of meditations basing on the method of practicing.

In meditations of the first type the attention is concentrated on signals coming from an object. We involuntarily practice it, when we narrowly look at something, attentively listen, sniff and intensively feel the pain symptoms or other sensations of our body. The most common of these meditations are *Trataka* — concentration of a look on the shining object, contemplation of the wood ball in China etc. Such meditations have two-sided effect. On the one hand, concentrating on an object we **actualise** it, i.e. consciously percept it, which widens our consciousness. On the other hand, long focusing can lead to distraction, caused by tiredness and **self-hypnosis**.

We can observe not only inner signals, but also people's stereotypes of behaviour. Here is an example from the Buddhist tradition.

Breathing in, one knows that one is breathing in; and breathing out, one knows that one is breathing out.

1. Breathing in a long breath, one knows, «I am breathing in a long breath». Breathing out a long breath, one knows, «I am breathing out a long breath».

2. Breathing in a short breath, one knows, «I am breathing in a short breath». Breathing out a short breath, one knows, «I am breathing out a short breath».

3. «I am breathing in and am aware of my whole body. I am breathing out and am aware of my whole body». This is how one practices.

4. «I am breathing in and making my whole body calm and at peace. I am breathing out and making my whole body calm and at peace». This is how one practices.

5. «I am breathing in and feeling joyful. I am breathing out and feeling joyful». This is how one practices.

6. «I am breathing in and feeling happy. I am breathing out and feeling happy». One practices like this.

48

7. «I am breathing in and am aware of the activities of the mind in me. I am breathing out and am aware of the activities of the mind in me». One practices like this.

8. «I am breathing in and making the activities of the mind in me calm and at peace. I am breathing out and making the activities of the mind in me calm and at peace». One practices like this.

9. «I am breathing in and am aware of my mind. I am breathing out and am aware of my mind». One practices like this.

10. «I am breathing in and making my mind happy and at peace. I am breathing out and making my mind happy and at peace». One practices like this.

11. «I am breathing in and concentrating my mind. I am breathing out and concentrating my mind». One practices like this.

12. «I am breathing in and liberating my mind. I am breathing out and liberating my mind». One practices like this.

13. «I am breathing in and observing the impermanent nature of all dharmas. I am breathing out and observing the impermanent nature of all dharmas». One practices like this.

14. «I am breathing in and observing the fading of all dharmas. I am breathing out and observing the fading of all dharmas». One practices like this.

15. «I am breathing in and contemplating liberation. I am breathing out and contemplating liberation». One practices like this.

16. «I am breathing in and contemplating letting go. I am breathing out and contemplating letting go». One practices like this.

The Sutra of The Full Awareness of Breathing

Second type of meditation is various forms of suggestion, i.e. active mastering body's functions by one's will. Depending on the way the volitional command is given, these meditations can be divided into visualisations, verbal and kinaesthetic suggestions. The most popular are first two of them.

During visualisation the command is done to subconsciousness in the form of some familiar visual images, pictures and figures. The most known is the visualisation of energy flow — as a shining with a certain colour; meditation on chakra's symbols, the inner organs, mandalas and so on. In verbal meditation a command is done verbally, like in a system of autogenic training by Schulz («My right hand is heavy and warm») and autosuggestions by E. Coue («I'm feeling better in all senses every day»). Practitioners of kinaesthetic suggestion try to provoke various sensations in their body (heaviness, lightness, warmth, coldness etc.) by a volitional effort.

The object of active influence in meditations of the second type can be not only physiological feelings, but also our thoughts.

«All thoughts, as soon as they are conjured up, are to be discarded, and even the thought of discarding them is to be put away».

Mahayana-Sraddhotpada Shastra

Meditation can also work with elements of one's worldview, with life position, identification and self-positioning in the world.

«He who practices 'clear observation' should observe that all conditioned phenomena in the world are unstationary and are subject to instantaneous transformation and destruction... He should observe that all that had been conceived in the past was as hazy as a dream, that all that is being conceived in the present is like a flash of lightning, and that all that will be conceived in the future will be like clouds that rise up suddenly».

Mahayana-Sraddhotpada Shastra

There is a belief that Western Psychology prefers active techniques, while in Eastern traditions prevail techniques of concentration, relaxation and contemplation, by which one can easily put himself into a state of delight, mind silence and trance. In fact this point of view is superficial. Every tradition had a broad choice of meditations of both types.

Considering all the foresaid, we should mention that only **meditations** of the third type are real meditations in the full sense of the word, and are a synthesis of both types of described exercises. Practitioner makes a volitional command to change his state, and at the same time is observing his state, which make it possible to control the effectiveness of commands and to adjust them, having more chances to achieve the wishful state.

Energy aspect of meditations

We considered meditations from psychological point of view. And what are they from the esoteric position? **Meditations are practices for the astral body.** Astral body like the physical one can be trained by special exercises, and the aim of this training, like with our physical and etheric bodies, is to make the respective body more **flexible,** i.e. able to reach a broader spectrum of states; **stronger**, i.e. more resistible to outer emotional influence; and more **energetic**, i.e. more vivid in its emotions. This means that meditations, like asanas, should be practiced in complex, with the clear understanding of your task and a plan of training, compensating one altered states of psyche by others, opposite ones — to make the range of possible states in real life broader, increasing degrees of personal freedom.

Sometimes the term meditation is significantly narrowed to some «calm», passive states of psyche. For example, the famous German researcher of yoga Dietrich Ebert defines meditation as «just a tropho-tropic state with the prevailing activity in parasympathetic part of vegetative nervous system». Nevertheless there are tens and hundreds of meditative techniques evidently shaking practitioner up, i.e. activating sympathetic branch of ANS. That's why we believe that this opinion is a reflection of the common misunderstanding of yoga in general, reigning in the Western world, which is a result of «religionizing» of many schools of Indian yoga. For more details about psychopractices see my monograph «Religious psychopractices in the history of culture».

FIRST STEPS IN HATHA-YOGA

Getting prepared

Meditating for actualisation

Before doing yoga (or any other things), you have to put yourself into a proper state.

Energetically a man represents a ball, or better say an oblong ellipsoid, but this ball can have many holes, punctures and energy outflows. In fact we go on arguing in some unfinished discussions, attach to some exterior objects, plan something for the future and regret about something already done. All these states cause outflows of energy, its «sticking» somewhere. There is a law of energy: «**Energy goes along with your thought**». So being physically in one place, energetically, emotionally (which is the same), we are at the same time in various places and situations. It is unfavourable in everyday life, because it weakens us, makes us less efficient; but especially dangerous this state is when we practice yoga. There is a principle I call «a principle of balloon»; if you puncture a hardly inflated balloon, the air will leave it slowly, but, if you puncture it well inflated, it may explode. Having energy holes and significant outflows, it makes no sense to practice yoga, because all the energy we pump during yoga session will immediately leak by our «tails». To avoid this, before starting we must liberate ourselves from such energy outflows, concentrating all our consciousness on ourselves and on the process we are in, to feel being «right here and right now». Like the octopus draws in its tentacles, we should keep all the energy to ourselves. «Gheranda Samhita» puts this technique this way:

> «As soon a Chitta, which is unsteady and has tendency to wander, exits the gate of feelings, you must harness it and put under control of Atman» (4.2.)

The **criterion** of a succeeded meditation is the feeling of warmth all over the body.

When you practice, especially when your body is significantly energized (remember the principle of balloon), your mind can leave the «here and now» again and wander somewhere else. Then the actualisation meditation should be repeated during the practice.

Padmasana
(lotus pose)

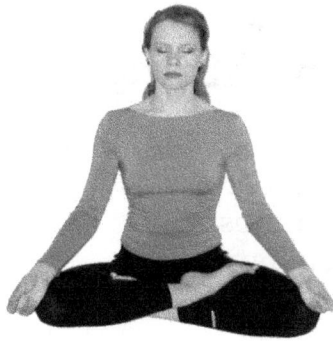

Arthapadmasana
(half-lotus pose)

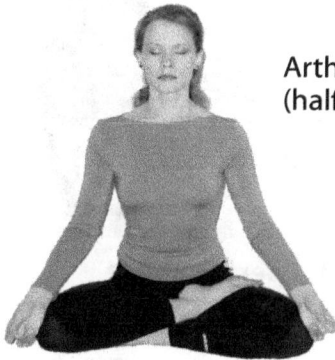

Siddhasana
(sidh pose)

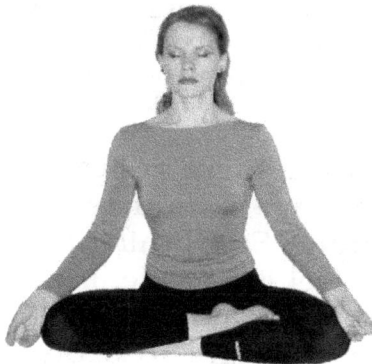

Sukhasana
(comfortable
pose)

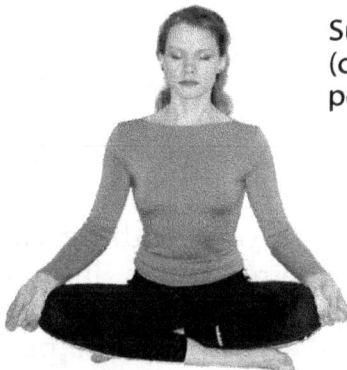

For meditation you must sit in one of the following meditative poses. **The crucial element is a straight back,** because we have a tendency to stoop at the level of depressed chakras, i.e. those zones, where there is an energy outflow. To avoid consolidation them by meditation, you must sit into a straight harmonious pose, even if in the beginning it may seem uncomfortable. By the way this discomfort can be used to actualise, by concentrating on it, your psychological problems that are causing it, and eventually start solving them (see the chapter «Meditation in yoga»).

Mentally pass all your chakras; if you see an outflow, take the energy back. Pass the Cosmos energy from the crown of your head along your spine down to the coccyx. Move your attention to the heart zone, smile by your heart to everyone present, to all living beings.

**Meditative poses
and mudras**

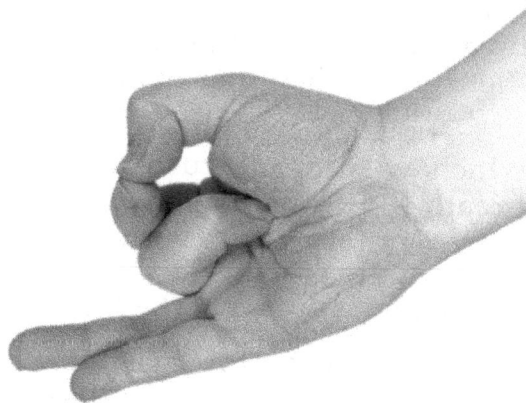

Djnana mudra

Full yoga breath
(rhythmical breathing)

They say «Eyes are the window to the soul». It is true, but in this case the second window to the soul is our breath. By the type and particularities of breathing you can tell almost everything about man's emotional sphere; and vice versa by changing our breath, we can significantly change our state.

Usually people **don't breathe by their problem zones.** If a person has a weak Manipura, he breathes only by the chest. If he has a weak Anahata, he breathes with the belly. If a problem zone is the solar plexus, he breathes with the «gap», somehow inhales with his chest and belly, missing one zone. If Anahata and Manipura cannot work simultaneously, then inhaling by the chest, we exhale by the belly. If Anahata's zone is blocked, we usually compensate it with Vishuddha — lifting the chest. The most awful breathing I call «spine breath», which is done by moving one's backbone — it is very harmful, because it breaks the heart's work. **The more superficial our breath is, the less respiratory muscles we use, the more problems we have.**

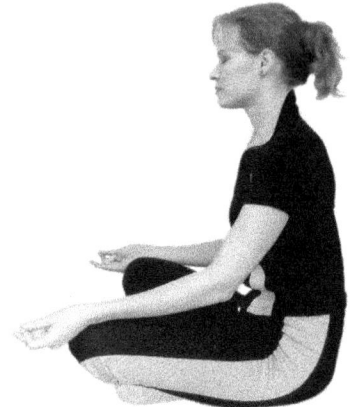

Faulty performance of Sukhasana
The spine is bent in the area of lower vertebrae. This carriage is often seen in cases of coccyx traumas. If it is impossible to sit straight, a thin pillow should be put under buttocks

The opposite is also true: **unblocking these zones, as well as respiratory muscles that were not used, we stimulate corresponding chakras and their psychological functions.** So learning to breathe with the chest, we learn how to love and to feel joy of life; breathing by our belly, we stimulate the sense of inner power and our social adaptation; breathing by the clavicles, we liberate our right to express ourselves, the right of the inner liberty.

Practicing yoga (except for special therapeutic techniques, about which we'll speak further) the best way to breath is with **full yoga breath** (FYB), also called **rhythmical breathing**. Such breathing activates all respiratory zones with no exception and in the right order, harmonising all chakras and providing the correct oxygen/carbonic acid ratio in the blood.

Some yoga origins claim that a slowed rhythm of breathing can significantly prolong our life, because a human being has a limited number of breathing cycles, so the slower he breathes, the longer time he can enjoy this resource. This statement is hard to prove, but psy-

54

chotherapists also have noticed such a pattern: the more serious is the patient, the more superficially he breathes. So the relation with the life duration is obvious.

Usually **mastering** FYB causes certain psychological difficulties. A man just does not notice that he misses some zones in breathing, from «inside» it seems to him that everything's all right. That's why before mastering full breath, we must perfectly master three auxiliary breathings, each of them having its important therapeutic effect.

1. Abdominal breathing, which goes from its name, is breathing just by the belly. To control it, you can put one hand on your belly and another — on your chest — it must stay completely still. Inhaling, the belly must stick out at the maximum, but not with the help of abdominal muscles — only by the air pressure. Exhaling, the belly sticks in as much as it can.

This exercise is supposed mastered, when you can breathe this way without much effort and discomfort, keeping the rhythm for at least five minutes.

> **WARNING!** The abdominal breathing lowers arterial pressure, so hypotension patients should be more careful performing this exercise. Hypertension patients can use it as a therapy and as an urgent self-aid, if they run out of meds.

2. Chest breathing is breathing with your thorax, just due to expansion of the chest and consequently widening of ribs. Most of modern people breathe harder by their chest, than by their belly, due to the blocked Anahata and the incitation to develop Manipura, more relevant to social realization, although just 20 years ago in the USSR the situation was contrary: people were easily breathing by their chest and could hardly master belly breath. At the Soviet times the strong Manipura was not just useless, but dangerous. Taking into account these difficulties, let's look at some details of performing this breathing.

First of all our ribs have several degrees of widening, of which we at the best usually use just one. Our thorax can be widened forward, by sides and up. **Mastering the chest breathing, it's better to check for activating all degrees of liberty, i.e. to widen the chest equally and extensively,** like a rubber ball. If your chest moves only forward or what is more often, entirely up, you should develop all missing respiratory degrees of freedom. By the way, psychologically breathing only «up» is related to the incapacity to express one's feelings, while «moving forward» tells that these feelings are insufficiently deep.

Some people find it difficult to «switch off» belly-breath, in this case they can use a belt or something of this kind to cord the belly in order to block the possibility to breathe by abdominal muscles. You can also ask for someone's help.

The common mistake is also to substitute the chest-breath for spine-breath: instead of widening ribs the practitioner moves ahead his entire thorax or strengthens his back, so that on the front view «it looks right». Of course all these are pathogenic types of breathing. To abandon this habit, you can practice breathing, lying on the floor or with your back pressed to the wall.

Like in the first case, the exercise is mastered when you can breathe like this with no discomfort or extra efforts, keeping the rhythm for about five minutes.

WARNING! Contrary to the belly-breath the chest-breath raises the BP, so hypertensive patients should be alert.

3. Clavicle breathing. Is done by the upper part of the thorax, due to its insignificant widening and stretching up.

The full yoga breathing is a combination of these three types of breathing.

Technique. Inhale by the belly, then by the thorax, then by the clavicles. Exhalation is done in the same order: from the belly, squeezing the ribs, dropping the clavicles.

Healthy respiratory muscular system

The main respiratory muscle is the diaphragm, with which other muscles cooperate: intercostal, pectoral, abdominal and shoulder girdle.

External intercostal muscles and anterior (interchondral) internal muscles are those of inhaling; posterior (interosseous) internal intercostal are the exhaling muscles. Muscles of the anterior abdominal wall — external and internal oblique and internal and external transverse and rectus are also exhalation muscles. Scalenes and sternocleidomastoids lift our thorax and set it, also working for inhaling. The same function can be done by trapeziform, pectoral and serratus muscle.

Recently another muscles' group role became clear — of the throat, tongue and soft palate. They receive an impulse, coming into a neurorespiratory drive some dozens of milliseconds before the impulse, going to diaphragm and pectoral muscles, providing by its contraction a normal potency of airways. We usually didn't consider them as respiratory muscles or muscles at all. Meantime just the soft palate has five groups of muscles, controlled by III, IX, X and XI pairs of cerebral nerves, forming pharyngeal plexus.

Inhalation is done by widening of the thorax in tree dimensions: lateral parts go up (increasing dextro-sinistral size), anterior part lifts (increasing the posterior-anterior size) and diaphragm goes down. At the vertical position men and women normally have a rib (chest) breathing, lying on the back — mostly diaphragmatic (abdominal).

Arbitrary change in the volume and speed, together with the effort, inhalation and exhalation — while talking, shouting, singing, playing musical instruments etc is usually done by diaphragm-abdominal breathing.

Respiratory muscle system also takes part in various actions, directly no related to breathing: in playing musical instruments, coughing, vomiting, defecation and others. The primary participation of these or others groups of respiratory muscles in these acts depends on its nature, the needed effort, body position etc.

Doing FYB correctly. After auxiliary breathings are mastered, the most common mistakes while practicing FYB are:

1. Inhaling by the chest you «blow off» the belly, pumping all the air to the chest. So the total volume of inhaled air significantly decreases. Such problem is typical for those who cannot live at the same time by Manipura and by Anahata, i.e. to use force, while loving and not hating a person, with whom they interact (needed, for example, for parents, punishing their kid not hating, but loving him). You should be careful not to decrease the volume of the belly at the rest of the inhalation.

2. Trying to breathe «with the spine», bending it when inhale and unbending at the exhalation. This is the most harmful way to breathe. To get rid of this custom, you should practice breathing in lying on your back.

3. Dropping the chest. After the inhalation is done, you should be careful to keep your respiratory muscles working, i.e. not to drop your ribs until you exhale by your chest. Otherwise your lungs will press the pericardial sac, hampering its work and provoking shortness of breath or even tachycardia.

4. Getting out of rhythm. The rhythm of breathing should be natural, i.e. easy to keep for quite long without any discomfort. Your natural rhythm is defined by the possibility to breathe without losing your breath. **The criterion of doing FYB right (as well as any other pranayama) is the fact that you don't need to recover your breath.** This breathing should naturally transform into your common breath. If you practice it regularly, your breathing cycle will become longer and you rhythm — slower, but it must be natural. In some yoga books it is recommended to practice breathing, counting till 8, 14 and even 30. This is fine, but it is reckoned on experienced yogins and can be harmful for beginners, because such a slow breathing may lead to breaking the rhythm (you'll wish to recover your breath after this practice), or even to malfunction of the cardio-vascular system.

5. Overtension in muscles. You should not make an effort at the end of exhalation.

You'll know that you are doing FYB the right way, if after 5-7 minutes of the exercise you feel warmth inside. Sometimes there is a light feeling of vibration or the even appearance of sweat, which also confirms, that the energy is activated in our body.

At the beginner's level start practicing FYB for 10-20 minutes a day, lying on something firm, before you go to sleep. It's important to do it on a firm surface in order to have a perfectly straight back, because when people start practicing yoga, they can hardly sit straight, and breathing in the curved pose would only secure a pathogenic posture.

After a month of such practice you usually become more energetic, start seeing bright dreams and sleeping better. In fact one of the signs of an increased energy are brighter dreams.

You mustn't do rhythmical breathing lying in your bed, even a very firm one, because it has its «sleeping» energy. When you sleep, a certain amount of your astral energy liberates and you get «switched» to some astral places where you go in your dreams, which hampers, when you practice exercises. That is why Pythagoras recommended to make one's bed — not from domestic, but from esoteric considerations. The bed should always be made after the sleep and better even hidden, because it keeps astral «switches».

Doing yoga you should always remember about your comfort, by the way like in any other occupation. **Caring about your comfort is a practice of Svadhisthana and Muladhara.**

Position of eyes during yoga practice

Where to look and at what to focus our look while doing yoga? Should our eyes be opened or closed? These questions appear from the first sessions, but to answer them correctly let's consult physiology and psychosomatics of the vision. Talking about the connection between our eyes and psyche, let's note the following.

1. Involuntary eye moves are caused by wandering of our mind. One of yoga's tasks is *dharana*, the stable state of mind. All psychosomatic processes are reversible, that's why the eyes can serve not only a great indicator of the state of our mind, but also a lever to influence it. In other words, if nothing else is previewed (like in the eye gymnastics) when you practice yoga, **your eyes should be motionless.**

2. There is an empirically proved interrelation between where you look and your state of psyche. A look below the horizon activates our subconsciousness, above the horizon — superconsciousness, eyes parallel to the ground — our consciousness. **Yoga is mostly aimed at development of our consciousness, so in most exercises the look should be zero-low.**

3. Maybe you»ve already noticed that when a person concentrates on his own problems, you can see it by a specific distracted look in his eyes, which become motionless and focus at the point 15-20 cm before his face. The look becomes empty. On the contrary, the image of a strong man is associated with the look into the distance. Indeed a point of natural eye focus is related to our capacity to extend our mind, to transcendent: the broader is one's consciousness, the easier he can look far to the horizon and keep this focus. Narrow-minded people can hardly look afar. The contrary is also true: wittingly keeping our look at the «eternity», helps to widen our consciousness. That's why practicing yoga, **your look should be focused at the «eternity»** (as if looking into the distance), if other isn't suggested. This focusing should be kept even if your eyes are closed.

4. Of course with closed eyes it is easier to digress from outer irritants. That is why when you start practicing yoga you should do all the exercises with your eyes closed, although then it is much harder to keep your mind stable. That's why at some point it becomes reasonable to practice with the open eyes. As for the experienced practitioner, it doesn't matter how to keep his eyes during the yoga class.

5. Remember that through our eyes we can receive or lose energy.

6. Some books recommend rolling up your eyes to focus them between the eyebrows. We can easily notice that whatever the position of the body, this focus inducts a specific euphoric high state, which is by mistake recognized as an effect from asana. Such state brings no good, it just distracts our consciousness from the body; that's why I strongly don't recommend doing it.

So in most exercises our look should be focused at the horizon[1].

In meditative poses you can often see a tendency to throw back your head, thinking that your spine is straight. If you throw back your head, almost all your muscles reflectively strain. No matter what happens, you should always reach the top of your head up and slightly forward.

---

[1]   Some sources call this eye position «vayshnavi mudra».

Orientation during yoga session

Most of Indian origins recommend doing exercises facing the North or the East. In ancient India these directions were sacred, but in other traditions, like esoteric qigong, we can find more complex approaches, relating orientation during the practice with your current tasks, seasons and even Moon phases, but even this approach implies outdoor practice where the natural electromagnetic field of the Earth is not distorted by man-caused influences. In the cities and condominiums with their reinforced concrete constructions, where modern yogins have to practice for the most of time, things are different. That is why the most favourable orientation should be found personally, guided by inner feeling.

«Set-ups» during practice

We can do exercises, including breathing, not only in different outside forms, but also with various «filling», which we'll call a «set-up» and correlate it with chakral system. For instance breathing with **Muladhara set-up** (Muladhara breathing) is a deep, heavy and dry breath. Besides inhaling, we stretch out respiratory muscles to the full.

If we make a graph of breathing, it would look like this.

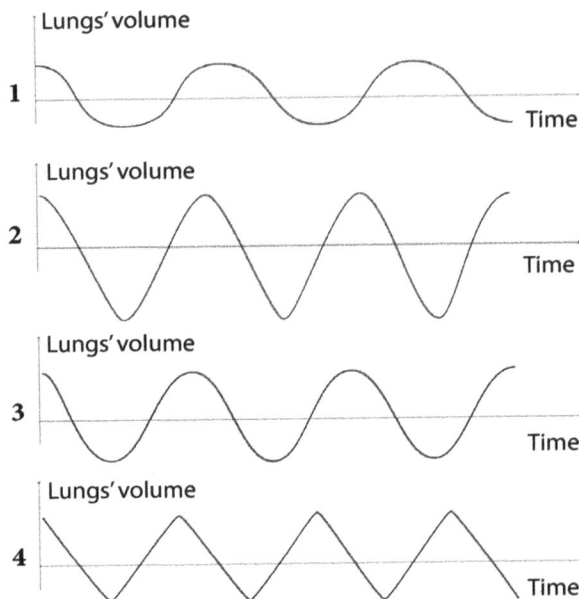

Graphs of breathing

1 — Anahata breathing;
2 — Manipura breathing;
3 — Svadhisthana breathing;
4 — Muladhara breathing.

Svadhisthana breathing is sinusoid: inhalation smoothly slips into exhalation and again to inhalation, so the speed of breathing changes. Respiratory muscles are not strongly involved — in Svadhisthana set-up you are not disposed to force yourself. Svadhisthana breathing is moist, warm, sometimes a little languid.

Manipura breathing is «angular», stiff dry and hot, like the runner's breath.

Anahata breathing has a more complicated structure, closer to a compact sinusoid. Such breath is warm and light.

«Svaradoya shastra» recommends another way of defining the type of breathing. You must close your passive nostril (see description of respiratory techniques), put a mirror to your nose and make several breathings. A figure formed by the condensate tells the type of your breathing: a square — for Muladhara, a half moon — for Svadhisthana, a triangle — for Manipura, a polygon — for Anahata, a round — for Vishuddha. It's quite exotic, but my observations proved, this method works.

Mastering the rhythmic breathing is better to start with the Muladhara set-up, because it helps to activate all respiratory muscles and to develop those of them that the person usually doesn't use. Besides this type of breathing strongly energizes our physical body.

Later you can breathe with different set-ups to activate and develop your chakras.

During natural human's bio cycle, which has a duration from 60 to 90 minutes, our breath passes all set-ups, from Muladhara to Ajna. It's the natural mechanism of chakra nutrition by prana of the air. Don't forget that this rhythm is related to the activation of one of our nostrils, corresponding to Ida or Pingala. This information can be used for selfish and unselfish ends. For example, when a person is breathing with Svadhisthana, you can make up to him at Svadhisthana, when he breathes with Anahata, use Anahata for the contact, and so on. Applying this knowledge to our personal training we should note that the most efficient way to work is to use your naturally activated chakra.

Warming-up

Warming-up is an important element of yoga complex. It is recommended before general exercises after completing hygienic procedures. Warming-up helps to activate our cardio-vascular system, increases flexibility, activates tokay of etheric energy. It is especially important for morning practices, because after a sleep all physical functions are slower and intensive routines at this time (including others than yoga, like jogging) can be compared to driving an unheated car, i.e. are destructive. **A warm-up should last not less, than 10 minutes,** because this is the time our cardio-vascular system needs to activate smoothly. Making your own complex, you can use just warming-up with no complicated postures just to warm up (for example, when you cannot freely move after an illness.

The warming-up should be done with Muladhara set-up, for it is the only way it can give the needed result.

The criterion to see, if you do it correctly is the feeling of heat in the active joint, which can be achieved only with Muladhara set-up. It means the proper *Grandha* is untwisted and the energy is flowing. If you feel nothing, nothing is happening.

Analysing how a person does his warming-up, you can diagnose almost all his problems, because by his posture he is unconsciously showing the state of his etheric body. For example, if a person has a depressed or breached Anahata, he involuntarily bends his elbows; if his Vishuddha is breached, he lifts his shoulders and strains his neck. Rotating the hips, a person shows his current energy state. If he has a problem with sexuality, the round is «cut» ahead, if he has many «tails», it's cut in the back part. If Svadhisthana doesn't work independently from other chakras, a person rotates all his body, being incapable to rotate just with one part of it. If Anahata and Svadhisthana move in opposite directions, it means they work anisochronously. The life position of such a man (of course, unconsciously) is «With the one we love we don't sleep, and those with whom we sleep life isn't much fun».

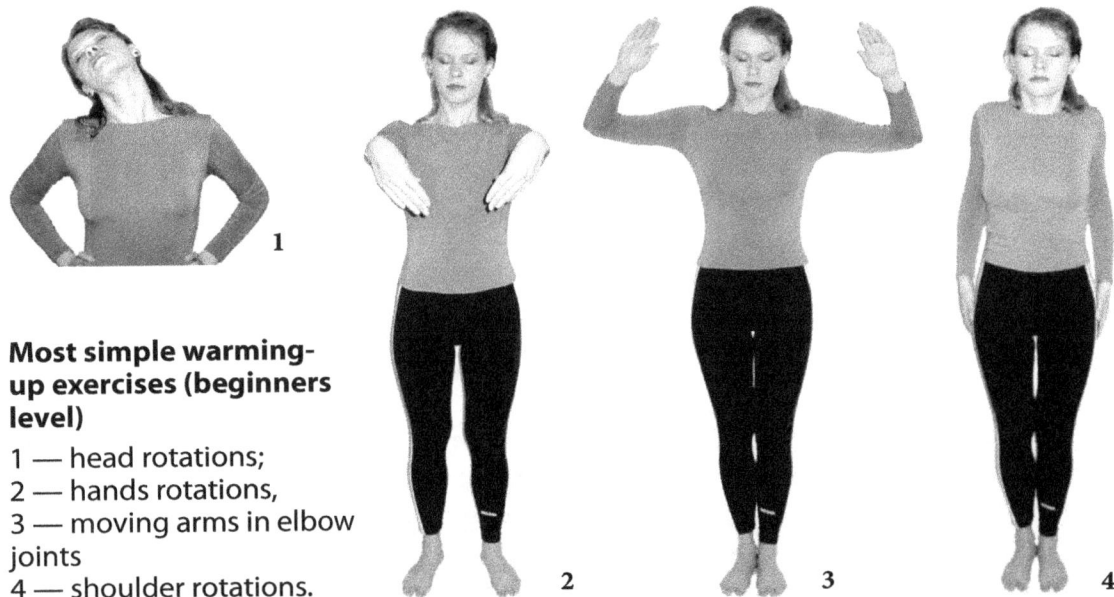

Most simple warming-up exercises (beginners level)

1 — head rotations;
2 — hands rotations,
3 — moving arms in elbow joints
4 — shoulder rotations.

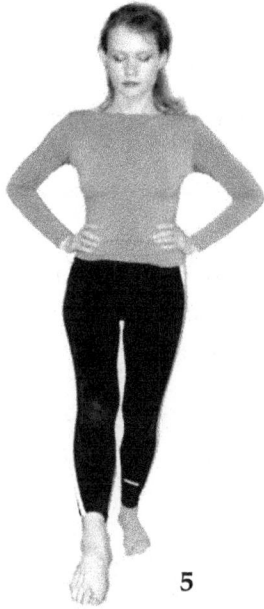

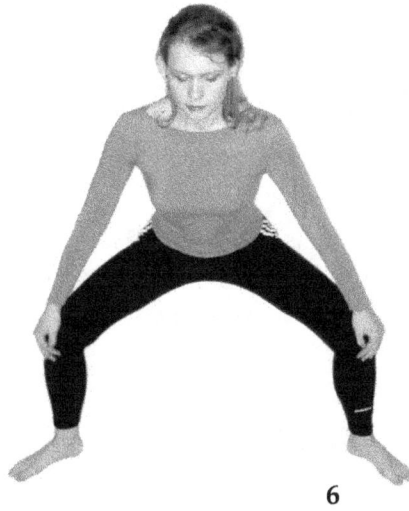

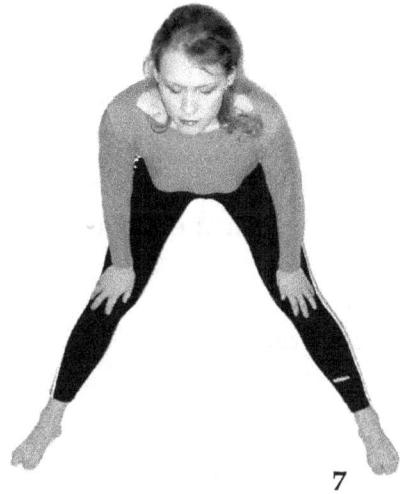

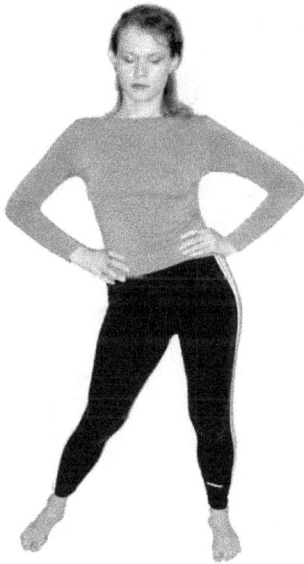

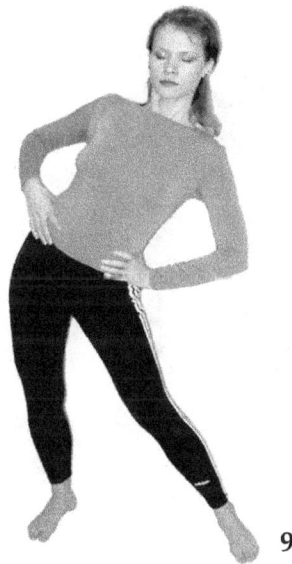

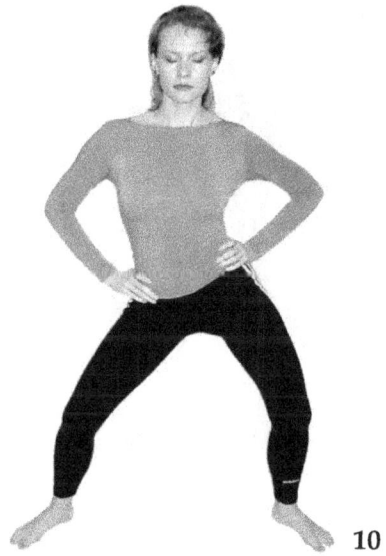

Most simple warming-up exercises (beginners level)

5 — feet rotations;
6,7 — warm-up for knees;
8 — pelvis rotation;
9 — rotation of pelvis together with torso;
10, 11 — pelvis rotation in squatting position.

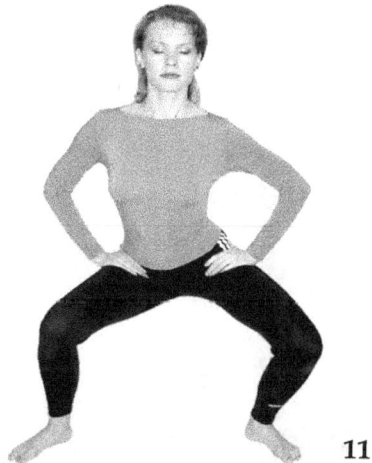

Dizziness and difficulties in getting the balance show that the consciousness is unstable.

The state of Muladhara can be diagnosed by the person's capacity to bend. If you can bend with your spine straight (just by your pelvis, with no bending in lower back) for more than 90 degrees Muladhara is integral.

At the beginners level it is better to do the warming-up with the Muladhara set-up. Doing exercises you should pay attention to the feeling of warmth in your joints. Every exercise should be done till the heat in the needed joint.

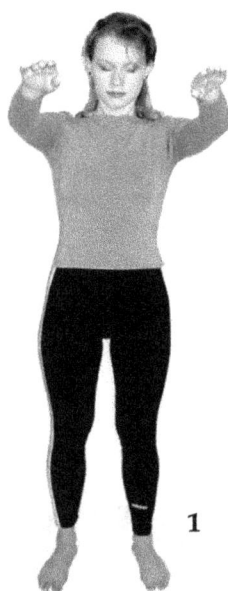

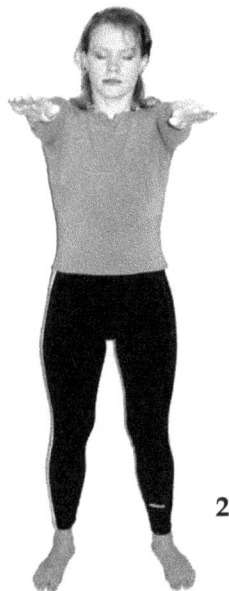

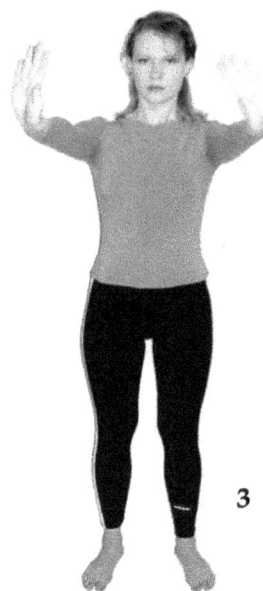

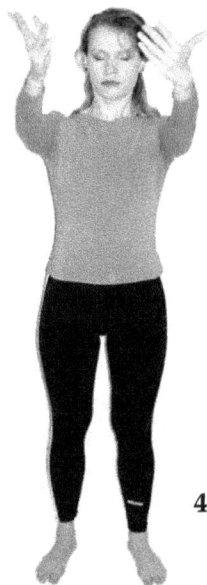

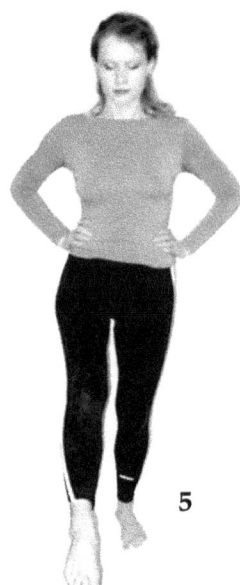

Mistakes in doing warm-up exercises (beginners level)

1 — arms are involuntarily folded in elbows (Anahata is breached or depressed)
2 — lifted shoulders cover the neck (indicates a breached Vishuddha)
3 — arms go apart (Anahata is over excited)
4 — energy «stuck» in Ajna
5 — hip goes ahead (indicates rigid Svadhisthana)

The most common exercises and general mistakes in doing them (beginners level)

Basic group of asanas

Bhujangasana (cobra pose)

Starting position. Lie on the ground face down, your head resting on your forehead or the chin, legs together, toes stretched out. The palms of your hands should be put on the ground slightly before your head, fingers extended, distance between hands about 20 cm. All the body, especially your shoulder blades relaxed as much as possible.

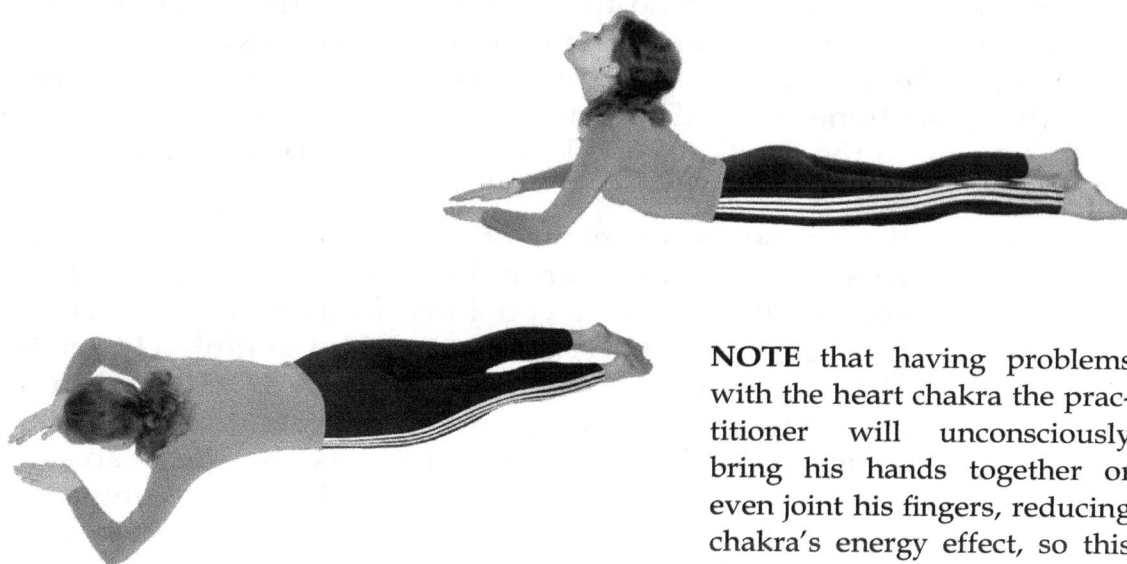

NOTE that having problems with the heart chakra the practitioner will unconsciously bring his hands together or even joint his fingers, reducing chakra's energy effect, so this should be watched.

Technique. At the exhalation do a slow backward arching with the spine, lifting vertebras one by one starting from your neck down to the lower back. Stay in the final position, breathing rhythmically. Going down is done at the exhalation, i.e. ending the position, we bring down, like a snake, by turns vertebra of the lower back, then of the thorax and of the neck, finally lying down the head.

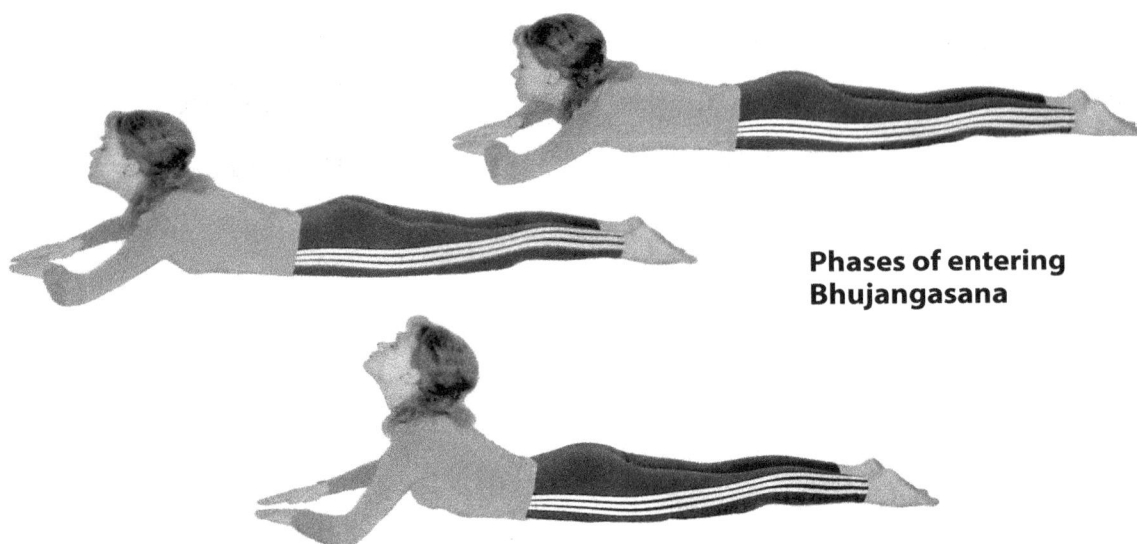

Phases of entering Bhujangasana

Particularities of performing. The feeling of a strained anterior-middle channel should move from the head down. Staying in the main part of asana, you should keep this strain long all the meridian. «Letting down» the tension at any part completely reduces to zero all the effect from the asana. Most often we take off the tension in the neck zone (the practitioner stops throwing back his head). In this case energy doesn't go up in the head and «sticks» in the shoulders, stimulating the development of osteochondrosis.

Here is **the energy mechanism** of this asana. Consequently entering asana we stretch our anterior-middle meridian[1], opening it. To open an anterior-middle meridian you have to stretch it so that the energy could flow in it, but it has to be **stretched completely (at the full length), gradually and successively.** The energy is gathered in the lower part of the body and after staying in the pose (when beginners start practicing yoga and still have «dirty» channels, the effect can come even after asana) it goes up the spine channel, **which is accompanied by the warm or even hot feeling moving up, to the head.** Such an effect from Bhujangasana is mentioned in «Gheranda samhita».

> «Fire of digestion in the body will rise intensively, all diseases will be cured and the snake-like Goodness (Kundalini) will wake up and rise thanks to practicing Bhujangasana» (2.43).

After asana the face and the ears can become red. The rising heat determines for how long you must stay in the posture.

---

[1]   Speaking about meridians we use Chinese terms, although those meridians by which energy flows, in yoga aren't completely the same as in Acupuncture, because the are located not on the surface, but deep in muscles. Nevertheless having no other elaborated terminology we'll use the closest one.

Every asana must be done till the needed energy effect from it is achieved. Staying in it longer is needless[1].

Exiting the pose, we close meridians, at the same time «smoothing» and returning the non-lifted by the anterior channel energy back by the posterior meridian. The understanding of energy mechanism explains the importance of entering and exiting the pose correctly. **The channel opens when it is stretched at all its length.** The block just in one place completely changes the energy picture of asana: the energy so to say sticks in the blocked zone, which can lead to unpleasant feelings and even provoke diseases. The most common mistake in entering this pose is not to lift the heart zone and after lifting the neck continue arching the lower back. As a result the energy doesn't go through the anterior channel and doesn't go up the posterior channel. The heart vertebra doesn't activate and the lower back vertebra gets traumatised because of the too zealous performance.

Mistakes in doing Bhujangasana

1 — buttocks are strained and lifted (energy get stuck in pelvis); 2 — no tension in the neck and thoracic spine (energy will get stuck in shoulders).

After this asana you should lie down for 1-3 minutes, practicing rhythmical breathing. As it was already said, the heat can go up even after doing the pose. Energy passes at a certain speed. **The «cleaner» your channels are, the faster energy passes.** When the beginner starts practicing yoga, his channels are quite «dirty», so that it takes up to 3 minutes for the energy to pass, but later this process can take some seconds.

The inner criterion of doing Bhujangasana right is the heat you feel, when the energy passes. After some practices there will be less heat, which means the asana can be intensified, for example, by putting your legs apart.

Initially you can feel other things than heat: pricking (like when your limb grew numb), chill, vibration, shivers etc. These sensations can appear when you start doing yoga and clean your channels (especially pricking, localized around the problem zone).

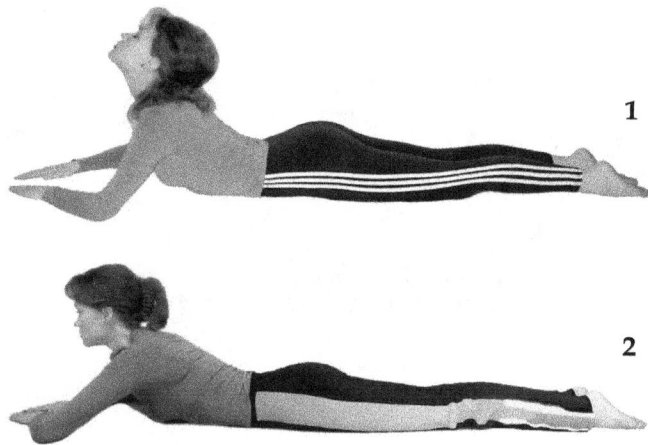

---

[1] This rule is true for beginners.

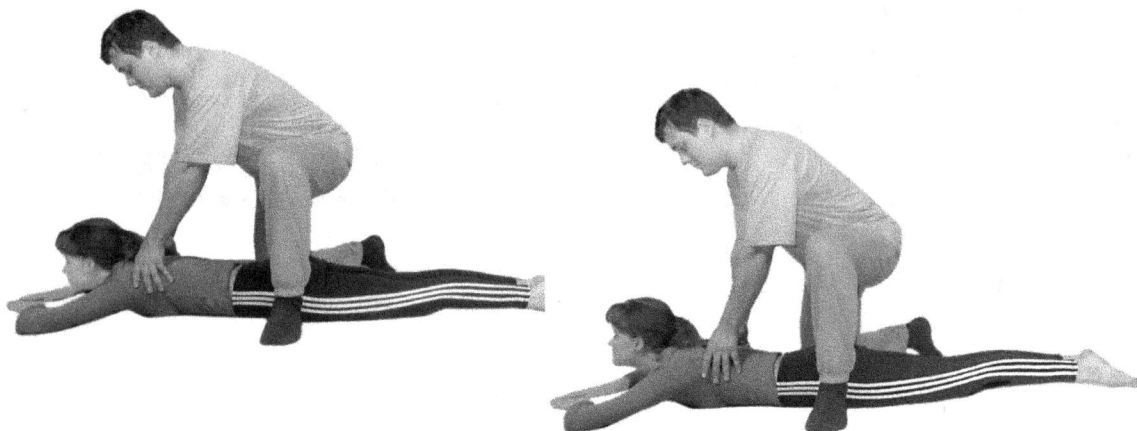

Making Bhujangasana with the assistant
The assistant immobilizes practitioner's back, preventing the tension
to «slip» problem zones in the spine.

It is important to do Bhujangasana **only** by longitudinal muscles of the back. Arms don't participate in this asana, to check for this try to lift your hands while being in the pose. In this asana **only** the foresaid muscles of our back are working, not those of legs, jaws, eyes, forehead, which can strain by reflex. Such correlations we call «pathogenic arches». In most cases these are stereotypes of movement, formed mistakenly and making people waste some energy for nothing. **To break down pathogenic arches — to master every group of muscles — is one of hatha's goals.**

Understanding how important it is to do asanas correctly, and that initially we tend not to notice our problem zones, it makes sense to start learning Bhujangasana and other basic postures with the help of another person, who'd control, if you enter and exit the pose correctly.

Every zone must be evenly activated. Your assistant can hold tight your spine with his hands, preventing the lower back from arching before the thoracic spine. He mustn't press, just set it. His fingers must stay on the muscles long the spine, not on your backbone. When a person lies relaxed it is easy to feel. Longitudinal muscles are relaxed when there is no tension and no contractions in them. If the practitioner goes up by these muscles (Bhujangasana isn't a push-up, it doesn't involve hands at all), all muscles long the spine are straining evenly bottom-up. Your assistant can feel, when the tension comes to his fingers, stop you in this position and move his fingers 2–3 dossals down. Then you continue arching and gradually come to the fourth vertebra. This way you breathe normally and should be controlled not to relieve strains in your neck — the energy will stop moving to the head and osteochondrosis can be provoked.

Pashimottanasana
(straining spine pose)

Pashimottanasana is a counter pose after Bhujangasana.

Starting position. Lie down on your back, feet together, hands long your body.

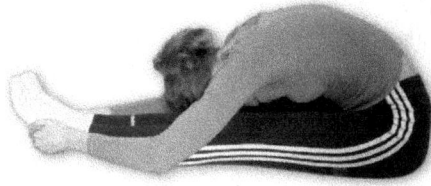

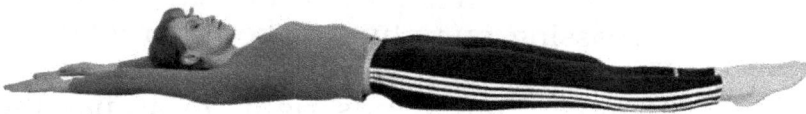

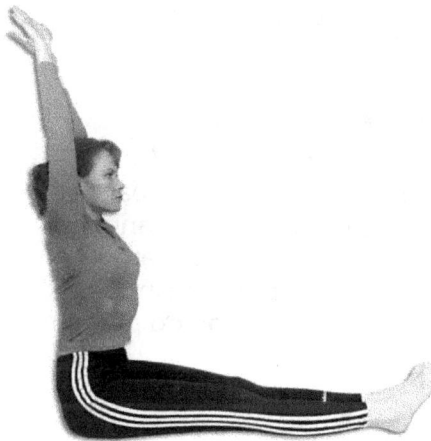

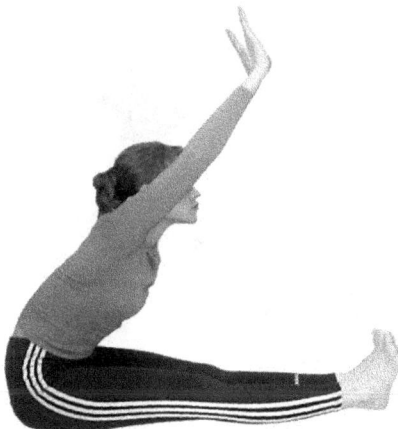

Phases of entering the asana

Technique. Inhaling to the full, stretch your hands above your head, stretch you body from fingers to toes. Exhaling, sit down, making 90° with your body, hands above the head, parallel to your upper body. Then as if someone is pulling you by the hands, bend ahead to your legs, starting from lower vertebra up the spine. Stay in this position, breathing rhythmically.

To exit this pose, do everything in the reverse order: from your head zigzagging, first stretch out your chin, arch with your chest, raise your torso and then lie down on the back. It is important to enter the pose this way, because we open our posterior-middle meridian bottom-up from toes to top, which means we must close it the same way — top-down. So we must exit the pose this way, «snake-like», as if entering Bhujangasana. **Exiting asana this way, we not only close our channel, but also stabilise the energy.** For example, you have brought some energy to the head — it will partly go down the anterior-middle channel, the rest won't make it. Not to have a heavy feeling in your head after doing this asana, we drive the rest of energy down the posterior-middle channel, exiting the pose «like a snake».

Particularities of performing. The feeling of tension in posterior-middle channel should move bottom-up. Staying in the static part of asana, you should **keep the tension long all the meridian: from top to toes.** Breaking in this tension closes the channel and brings to zero all the effect from asana. In addition to making energy move, this pose can also activate etheric tockays in the **external field**, i.e. in the outer part of our etheric body, surpassing our physical body, around us. The first clue to work with this energy is to move your hands right. In asanas the etheric energy follows the hands. So hands must always be straight and strained.

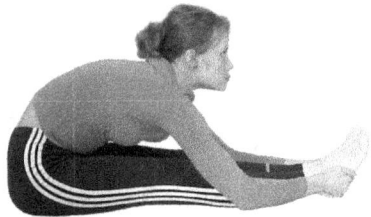

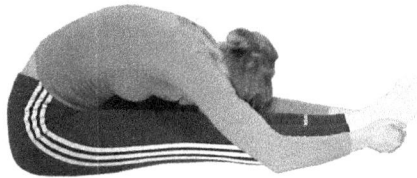

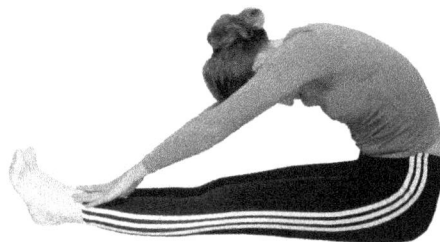

PICTURES Phases of entering the asana

Mistakes in doing Pashimottanasana

No tension in lower back and buttocks, energy channels in legs are not activated. The excessive bending in thorax can lead to raised blood pressure.

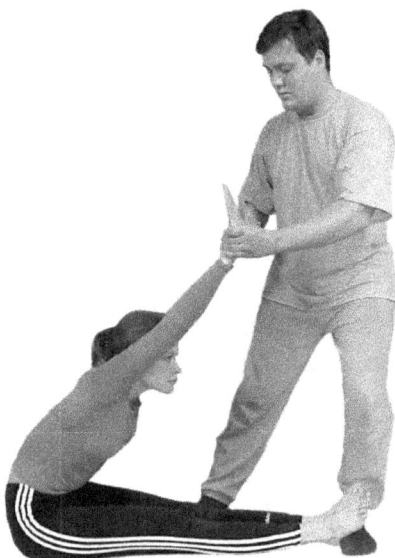

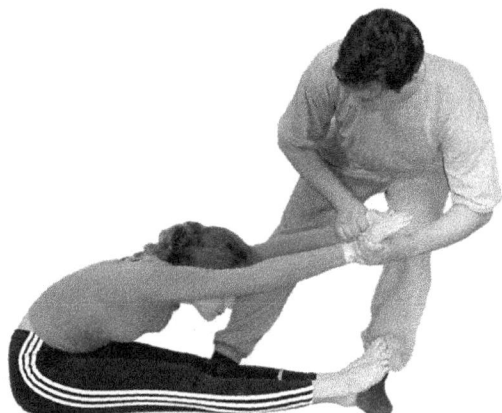

Doing asana with an assistant
Assistant pulls by hands, providing even tensioning of the back

70

Vakrasana (curved pose)

Vakrasana is one of the local-stretching squeezing poses.

Starting position. Sit on the floor.

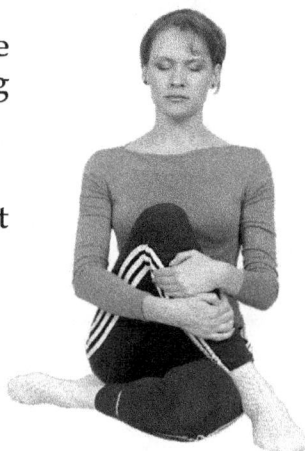

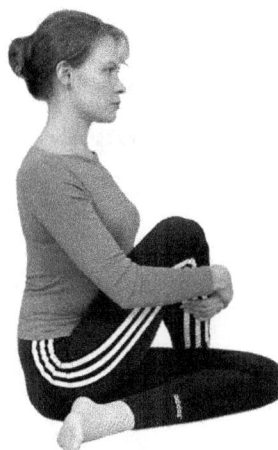

A simplified variation of vakrasana

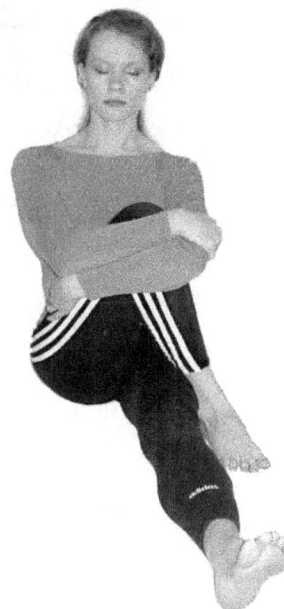

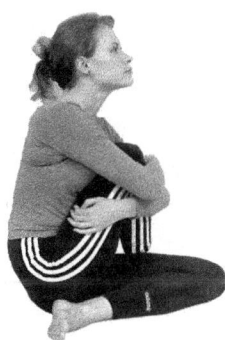

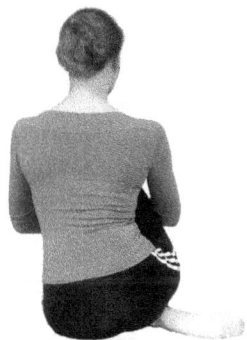

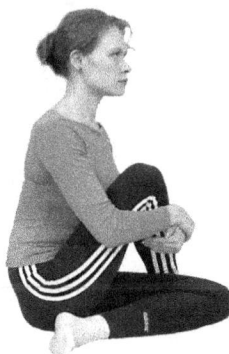

Technique. Put one foot to the opposite buttock (as if entering the lotus). The other leg bend in the knee and put over the opposite hip, the foot parallel to this hip. The back is straight and perpendicular to the ground. The shoulders are at one level, both buttocks — on the ground. Slowly pull the knee to our chest to feel the strain in the buttock. Pain in the buttock is explained by a non-realised sexual energy, which we assign to our body.

Particularities of performing. You shouldn't crook to the knee or pivot to reach it. The posture must be absolutely straight.

Mistakes in doing Vakrasana

1 — the lower back is crooked (no tension in a buttock); 2 — one of the buttocks doesn't touch the ground (energy gets stuck in the kidney); 3 — not the knee is reaching the body, but the body goes to the knee.

71

Arthamatsiendrasana
(pivoted spine pose)

Starting position. Vakrasana.

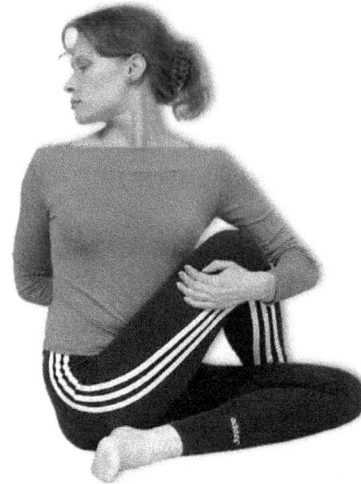

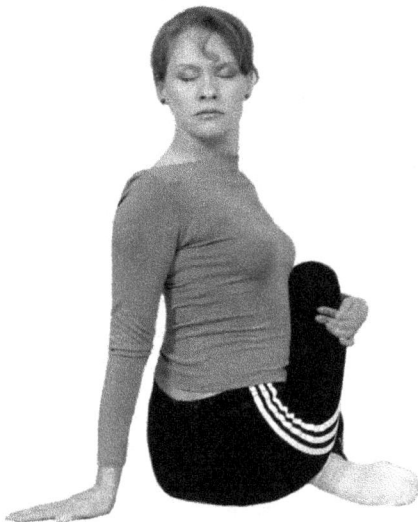

Technique. Pivot your spine in the direction of your upper knee, to rest on it. Your back must stay absolutely straight, shoulders at the same level. Don't lift your buttocks off the floor. Pivoting must be even — from coccyx to upper cervical vertebra.

Particularities of performing. You should achieve a **feeling of even tension-pivoting of longitudinal muscles of your back: from the head to the coccyx.** In this asana the spine must be perfectly straight and perpendicular to the ground.

Arthamatsiendrasana is a very efficient pose in treating osteochondrosis and scoliosis, but on conditions that it is done correctly, i.e. with the straight back. If these conditions are not fulfilled, the performance of asana can worsen these diseases.

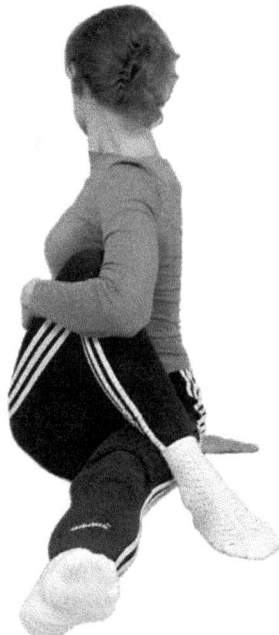

A simplified variation of Arthamatsiendrasana

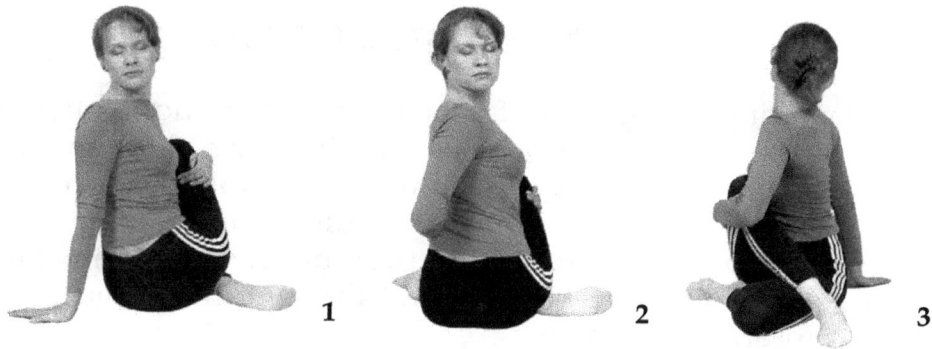

Mistakes in doing Arthamatsiendrasana

1 — one of the buttocks is off the floor;
2 — no pivoting in lower back (energy goes up not from buttocks, but from Manipura);
3 — head is thrown back (energy blocked in the neck); 4 — S-formed spine (tension from pivoting is lessen, energy dispersed in the back); 5 — the crooked back (such performance causes microtraumas in intervertebral disks and provokes osteochondrosis)

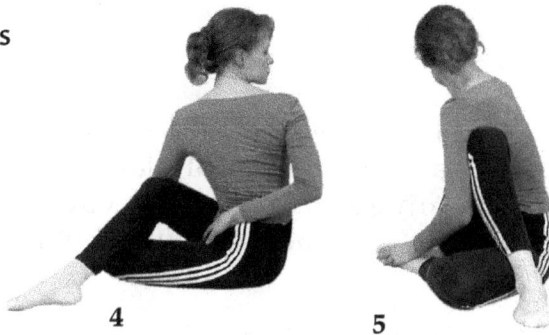

This is a completely balanced complex for beginners. To do it thoroughly and with no hurry, it takes about 15 minutes. You should never hurry to do exercise and learn to take pleasure from every asana. This complex cleans main meridians and drives energy by the main round, which can be correlated with the microcosmic orbit in Chinese tradition. If you practice at your own, you can do this complex during one month. After that you'll become used to these exercises, and the effect from asanas will diminish. In this case (and only in this case!) you can (and should) widen this complex and add some more complicated asanas.

When people start practicing yoga, they can get agitated (especially, if they feel an effect from asanas): they want to practice more, to do more asanas etc. It is the wrong way. Firstly passionate desires burn out quickly, secondly the amount of energy you can accumulate during one yoga session is limited by the capacity of your chakras. In a one-litre jar you can put only one litre of water. With time and practice this volume will increase together with the energy potential of the practitioner. At this point you can spend 40–50 minutes doing yoga, including hygiene, warming-up and rhythmical breathing before going to sleep — it will be enough. The hurry is a state where our energy runs before us, to the future, that's why we can't reach it. We should work with ourselves gradually without violence.

Second group of asanas

Mastering this group of asanas should be done after having mastered asanas of the first group, as well as when the physiological effect from them diminishes (there is no more physiological sensation of heat). In the yoga complex these asanas should be done after the postures of the previous group, because they provide the more intensive «untwisting» of energy as for its density and the length of trajectory (activating channels in arms and legs).

Ushtrasana (camel pose)

As for its action and technique, this asana is similar to Bhujangasana, but it is «more powerful», because it uses gravity and activates the hips.

Starting position. Take an on-knee position «Japanese-like», feet on toes, hips open at 15 degrees (in yoga this position is called «vadjrasana»).

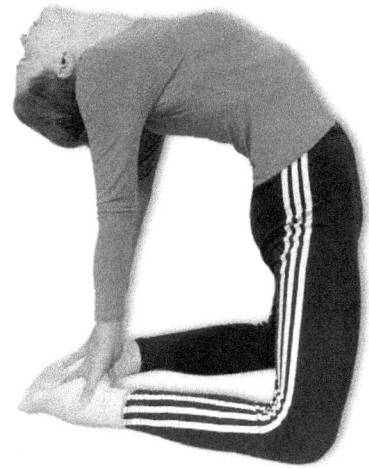

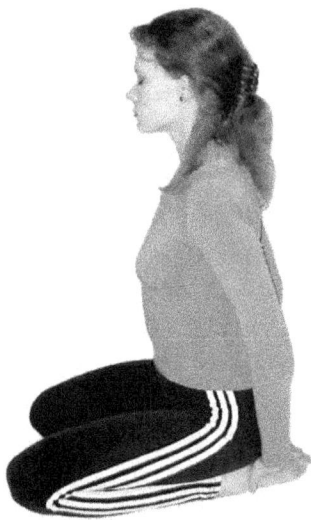

Technique. Inhaling, arch in the spine, starting from upper vertebra, like in Bhujangasana, gradually stretching out anterior-middle meridian. At last stick ahead your pelvis, grab your heels by your hands and rely on them. Exit exhaling in reverse order, straightening yourself bottom-up, vertebra per vertebra.

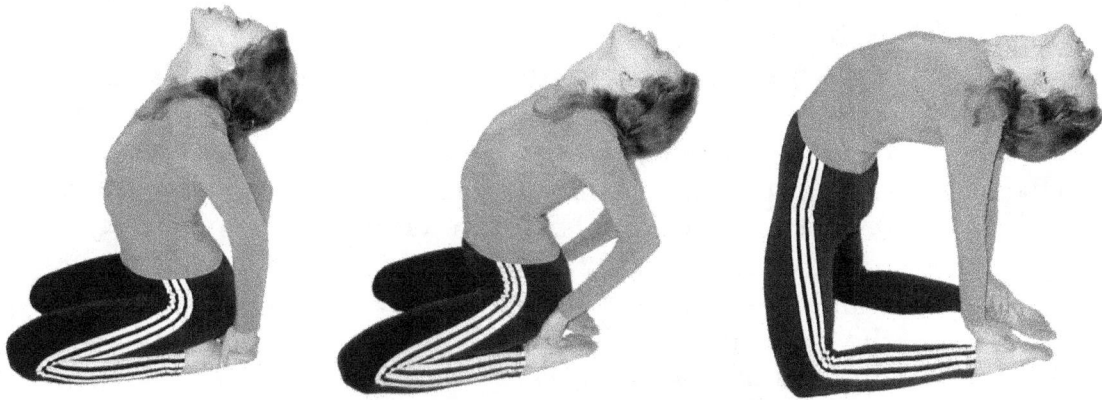

Phases of entering Ushtrasana

Particularities of performing. In the static position of asana pelvis and knees should be in one line. Avoid «sharp turns» in the spine. **The tension must be evenly distributed from the knees to the chin.** Those who have blocks in the anterior part of their hips (which indicates that their Svadhisthana is clogged) find it more difficult to do this asana, but this practice can help them to release the block and to liberate the non-realised sexual energy, which tends to accumulate in the anterior part of the hips. For men this asana can help with the problems of premature ejaculation.

Padahastasana
(pose of feet to hands)

This asana is similar to Pashi-mottanasana, only done in standing position.

In Padahastasana the energy goes not only due to the bending, but also due to the gravity, influencing the blood, intensifying the humoral effect. So padahastasana is to some extent an inverted pose.

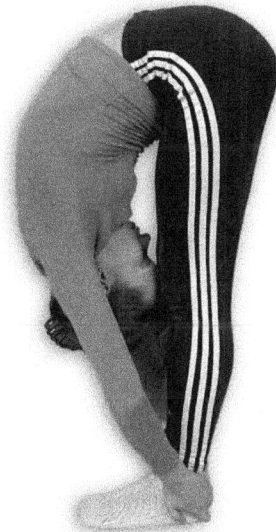

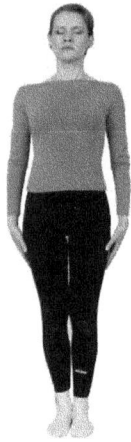

Starting position. Stand straight, legs and feet together.

Technique. Inhaling raise your straight hands, exhaling bend your body ahead and down, vertebra per vertebra starting from the lowest ones. Put your hands on the ground near the feet or on your calves and pull your body to your legs, stretching your spine. Try not to bend your knees. Exit asana with an exhalation, «like the snake» — starting from your neck bones. While exiting the pose, hands glide freely long the body, as if «smoothing» your etheric body.

Particularities of performing. The posterior-middle meridian must be evenly stretched and felt long all your back — from the heels to the head. Control your spine to be bent evenly.

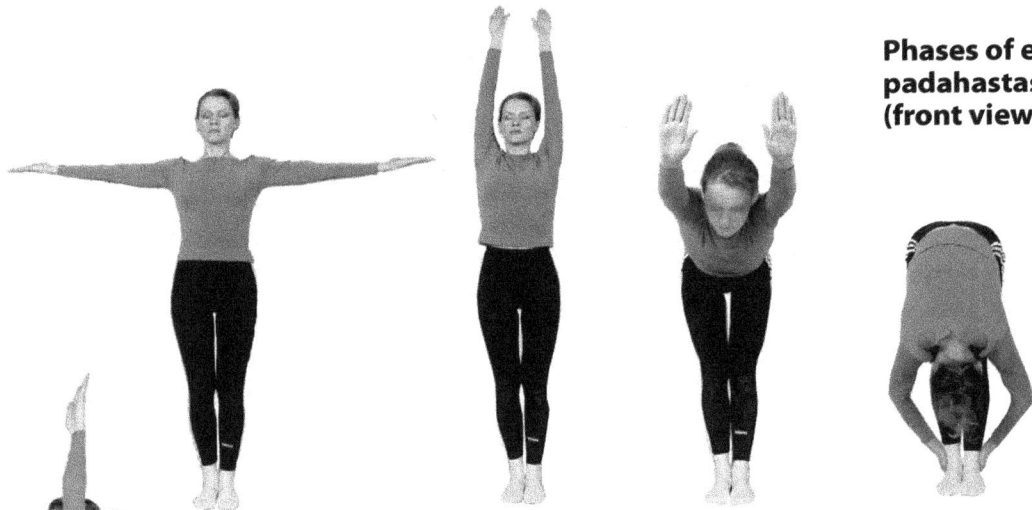

Phases of entering padahastasana (front view)

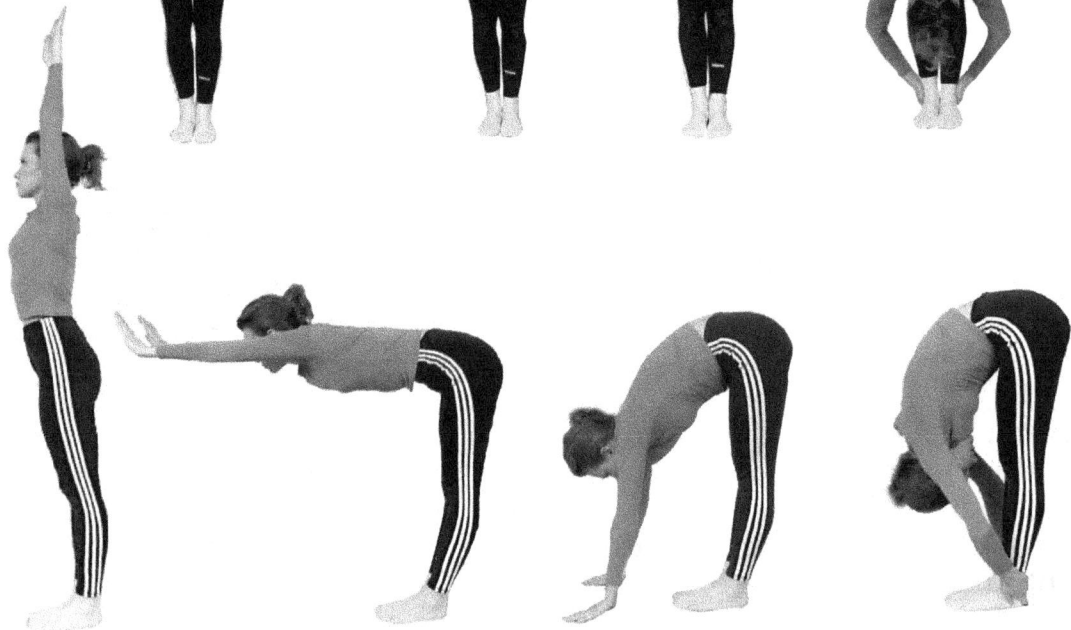

Phases of entering padahastasana (side view)

76

Trikonasana (triangle pose)
Simplified version

Starting position. Stand still and straight, feet parallel, one and a half shoulder width apart.

Technique. Inhaling, raise your hands by your sides to the level of your chest. Exhaling, simultaneously pivot your body bottom-up and bend ahead with your hip joints. **Your back must remain straight, pivoting vertebra after vertebra**. Don't crook your spine, neither change your pelvis position (throw it aside), otherwise asana will cause only harm. Men should start pivoting to the left side; women — to the right side. Face and look are directed up, to the risen hand. Breathe rhythmically. Exhale and inhaling start untwisting from your head and raise your body. Put your hands down. Repeat for the other side.

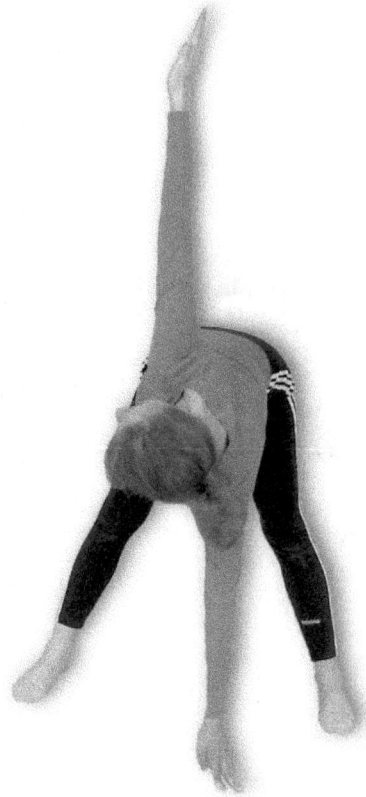

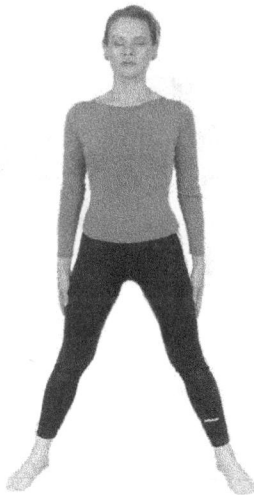

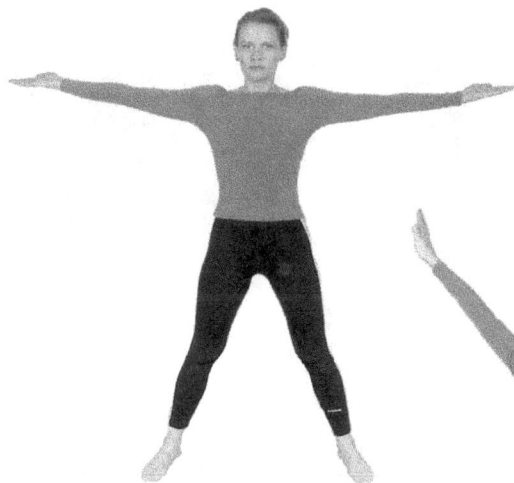

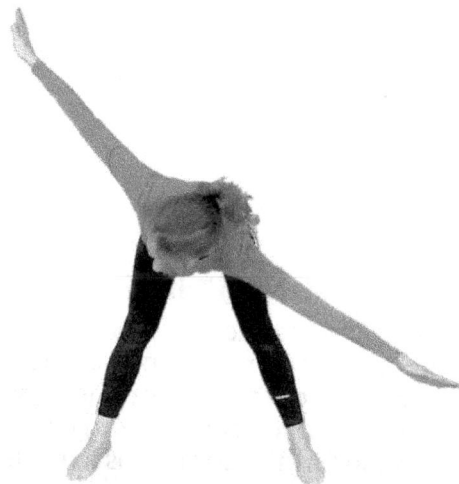

Phases of entering Trikonasana

Phases of entering Trikonasana

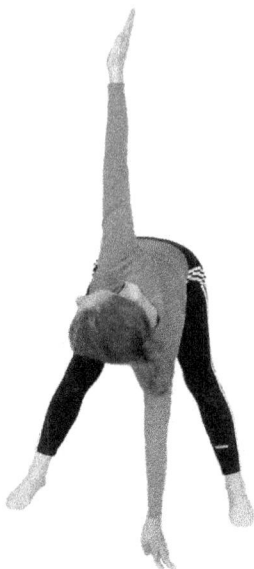

Particularities of performing. Pivot the straight back and don't shift your pelvis. The spine should be twisted evenly. When you do this asana, your legs and pelvis don't displace; pivoting and bending the body should be done simultaneously, keeping your back straight. Too much energy is equally harmful as lacking it. When you do an asana, a part of energy is consumed by your organs and partly it is felt as the warmth or the heat moving in your body. Trikonasana acts like an enema: energy squeezed from your pelvis due to pivoting, goes up the anterior-middle meridian, which is opening thanks to gradual pivoting. Seeing the mechanism of the asana, you can understand criteria of doing it right: pivoting should be done bottom-up, so that the squeezed energy could rise.

The inner criterion of doing asana right is the feeling of the heat, rising spirally up to your head.

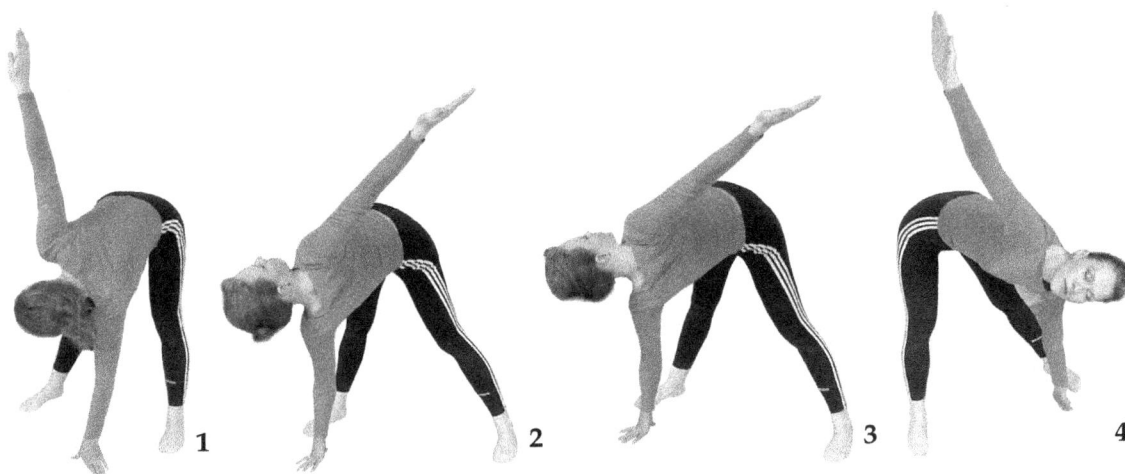

Mistakes at doing Trikonasana

1 — doing the exercise with the stooping, not pivoted back — channels don't open. It's the most common and harmful for health mistake; 2 — shifting the hip: energy isn't squeezed from the buttock up, but goes down to the hip; 3 — the same, plus inclining the head, which blocks energy in the neck; 4 — back is pivoted not from the coccyx, but from the fourth vertebra, as a result energy cannot pass the lower back. Head is thrown back — also a current mistake

Final group of asanas for beginners

Dhanurasana (bow pose)

Starting position. Lie on your belly, bend your knees and grab your ankles.

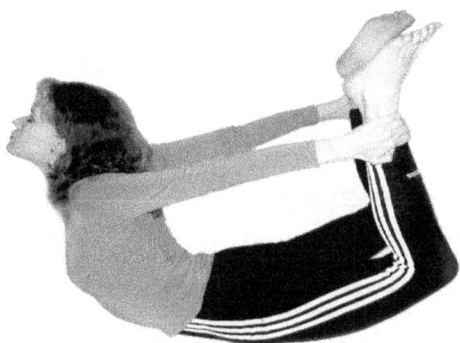

Technique. Inhaling, arch back, raising your upper body and your legs. **The angle of ascent of the legs and the upper body should be the same. Relax all the not involved muscles.** Exhaling, let go your ankles, gradually straightening your body — from the lower back up and down.

Particularities of performing. Watch the even tension in your anterior-middle meridian. If the rhythm of your breathing breaks, decrease the angle at which you raise your body. By the breathing your body can rock, but don't do it expressly. The angle of ascent of your legs and the upper body should be almost the same.

Inner criterion — feeling energy (heat) flow to the point of contact with the floor.

Mistake at doing dhanurasana

Legs are raised less than torso. Such performance isn't harmful, but the effect from asana will be minimum

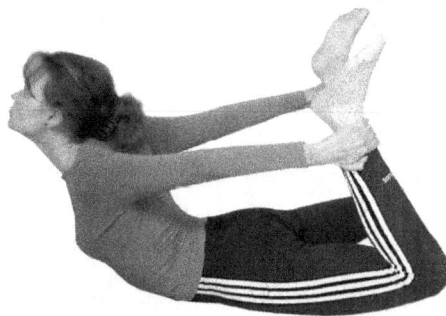

Halasana (plough pose or love pose)

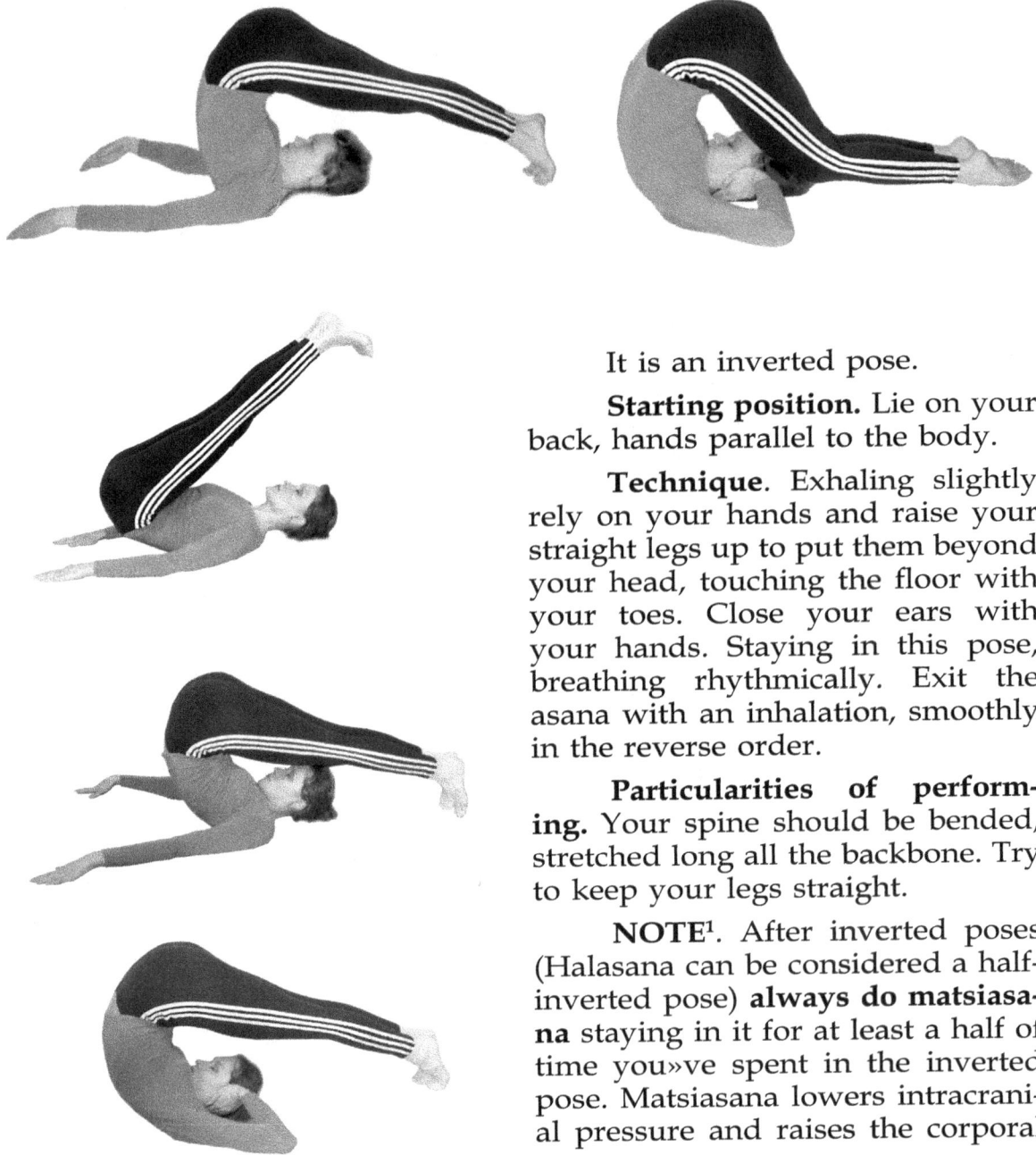

Phases of entering halasana

It is an inverted pose.

Starting position. Lie on your back, hands parallel to the body.

Technique. Exhaling slightly rely on your hands and raise your straight legs up to put them beyond your head, touching the floor with your toes. Close your ears with your hands. Staying in this pose, breathing rhythmically. Exit the asana with an inhalation, smoothly in the reverse order.

Particularities of performing. Your spine should be bended, stretched long all the backbone. Try to keep your legs straight.

NOTE[1]. After inverted poses (Halasana can be considered a half-inverted pose) **always do matsiasana** staying in it for at least a half of time you»ve spent in the inverted pose. Matsiasana lowers intracranial pressure and raises the corporal pressure.

---

[1]   This doesn't concern advanced yogins who construct their complex according to a more complicated principle.

80

Matsiasana (fish pose)

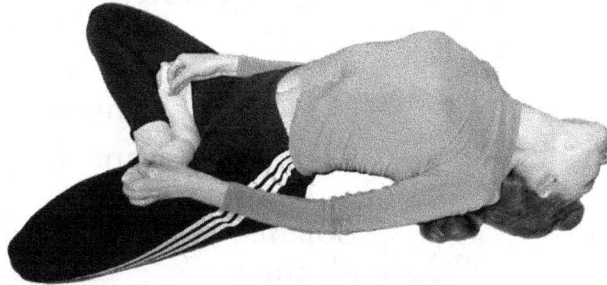

Starting position. Sit in the lotus, half-lotus or sukhasana (with your legs crossed).

Technique. Throw yourself back and put the top of your head on the floor. The head should be thrown back to stretch your anterior-middle meridian. Especially it's important to stretch the anterior zone or your neck. Let your shoulders go back at the maximum. Breathe rhythmically. Exit in the reverse order. Asana is done for 1-2 minutes, but not less than a half of time spent in the inverted pose.

Particularities of performing. When you stay in this pose, it's especially important to relax your muscles of the back of your neck. Only in this case asana makes the venous blood flow out of your head. The additional influence of this asana has to do with the blood flowing to your thyroid, liberating hormones from it, «sitting» there in their follicles. As a result during a correct performance there is an increasing trembling all over your body and a heat.

Matsiasana (simplified versions)

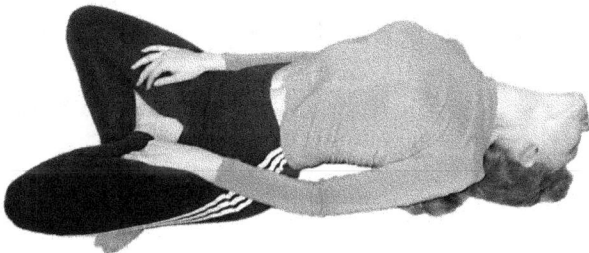

1. Enter the pose from lying position. Exit the same way.

2. Don't cross your legs, rather bend your knees and put your feet as close to your buttocks as possible. Bend as described above.

Sarvangasana
(overall pose or the pose for all parts of the body)

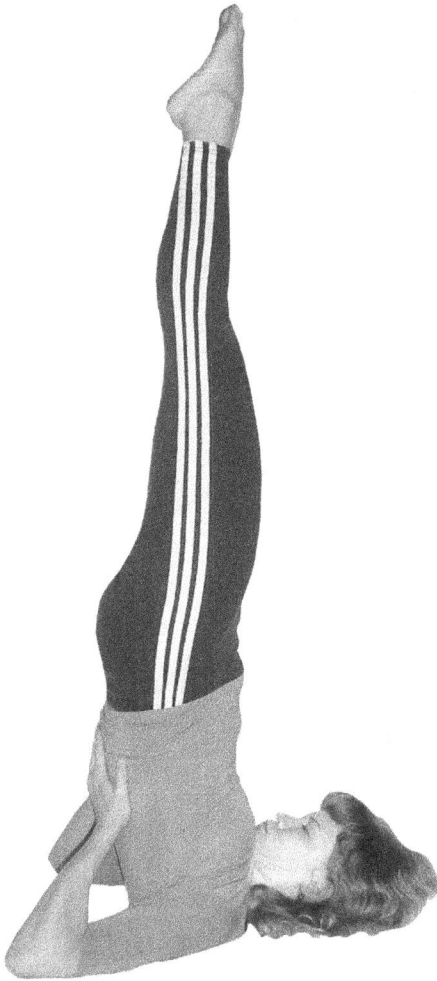

This is an inverted pose.

Sarvangasana is not difficult and can be done by anyone, who has no problems with his spine — especially with the neck.

Technique. It is performed by first lying on the back with hands under the mid-back, then lifting the legs and lower body so that the weight of the body is supported on the head, neck, upper back and upper arms. Breath is rhythmical. Entering and exiting the pose must be slow. If you have problems with your spine, or, if your neck is weak, it can be done not vertically, but at 45-60 degrees to the ground, holding the body with your hands.

How it acts. This position of the body stimulated the blood flow in the vertebral artery to the back of the head, stimulating all centres in visceral regulation brain streams, improves functioning of all viscera and all the body's performance, that is why it is called «posture of the complete body». It is a good preventive measure from varix, helps, if there are disorders in cerebral blood flow, but first of all this posture favours functioning of the left ventricle of the cardiac muscle. This asana efficiently replaces aerobic exercises, strengthening your heart.

Pranayamas

Common remarks about pranayamas

We should proceed to pranayamas after having practices asanas for some time. Indeed pranayama's goal is to energize and fix the energy structure, after it was purified and formed by asanas. If this structure is absent, pranayamas can blight you. Besides, to do pranayamas correctly you must feel your body in the more subtle way. Doing pranayamas inaccurately, you can have more unpleasant consequences, than after practicing asanas. Usually pranayamas are done after the complex of asanas (for beginners I recommend only this order), but the «mixed» complex can also be done — alternating asanas with pranayamas at a certain scheme (see chapter «Principles of building a yoga complex»).

All pranayamas must be started with a deep (as deep as possible) exhalation. Physiologically it is explained by the fact that in our lungs there is a so-called «middle column of air». When we exhale, the exhausted air from bronchus and alveolus goes to it; and when we inhale, the fresh air mixes with the air from the middle column. This mix goes to active parts of lungs, reducing efficiency of breathing. The maximum exhalation is needed to take away all the exhausted air from our lungs.

Kapalabhati (cleaning of the skull)

Kapalabhati is the rhythmic breathing done by the belly with the speed of 90120 breathings per minute. Ratio of inhalation and exhalation duration is 3:1. Number of breathings per minute is individual and should be defined by achieving the greatest effect. Beginners (especially with not trained diaphragm breathing) should do about 60 breathings per minute, and then increase this rhythm.

The main mistake in doing Kapalabhati is to use pectoral muscles, which can lead to «break-ups» of heartbeat and cause pain in the diaphragm.

How it works

1. Physically Kapalabhati is an intracranial hydraulic massage of the brain, done by pressure difference made by the belly.

2. Keeping a certain rhythm, we change the ratio of oxygen/carbonic acid content in our blood, in this case — by increasing the content of oxygen[1].

3. In human's nose there are special nosehairs, directly related to our brain. Rhythmically influencing them, we stimulate our brain.

The inner criterion of doing it right is the feeling of «enlightenment» in the eyes after doing pranayama, as if the room became clearer, which probably gave pranayama this name.

---

[1]   Unfortunately I ignore researches where the exact correlation would be defined, nevertheless such a liaison and some regularities can be noticed empirically.

Akahalabhati

Akapalabhati is a similar pranayama, only that the inhalation is done by both nostrils and exhalation — by one, changing it every time. Nostrils are closed by the right (for men) and left (for women) hand, performing yoni-mudra (middle and index fingers are pressed to the base of the thumb around the line of life, other fingers are straight).

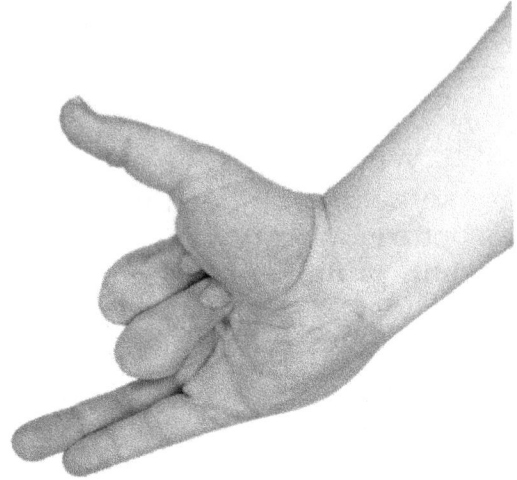

Yoni mudra

How it works. Akapalabhati works the same way as the previous pranayama, but because of reducing the permeability of the air in inhaling, the hydraulic wave is twice stronger, that's why the effect is greater.

Another mechanism of action has to with the altering stimulation of Ida and Pingala, widening the spectrum of ANS states.

Ujaya (victorious)

Ujaya is an exercise, by which we do an internal massage of the endocrine glands. These glands are located deep in the body and have no mechanic access, so they are massaged by vibration. Human being is like an acoustic resonator of voluntary volume, which helps to focus vibrations on each gland, one by one, changing the pitch and the frequency of sounds.

Ujaya is a successive singing of sounds, forming a sacred mantra **OM**, which can be decomposed to some sounds: **Ah, O U, M**. Every sound is related to a certain zone and resonates in it. Sound «A» should be sung to feel the resonance (physical feeling of vibration, tickling) in the upper fornix of the skull, «O» — in the part of the third eye, «U» (like in «who») — in sternum, «M» in Muladhara. Ideally sounds should follow with no break, so that the vibration would pass from the crown of the head to the groin.

If needed you can stimulate some chosen glands, singing just a part of the mantra. Actually ujaya can be done by other mantras, if you can diagnose their effect and know which effect you want to receive.

WARNING! Ujaya makes a strongly pronounced stimulating effect, so don't abuse this exercise.

Kumbhaka
(holding breath after inhaling[1])

This exercise can be done either separately or together with other, more complicated exercises. Its action is based on the accumulation of carbonic acid, which results in general toning of the body.

Technique. Inhale by FYB. Hold your breath, closing tree bandhas. Exhale, unlock bandhas.

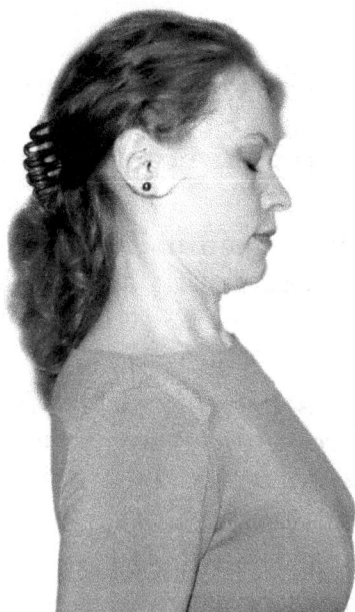

Particularities of performing. Inhaling, respiratory muscles cannot be relaxed until the exhalation is done. This detail — a need to hold the thorax open — is fundamental, because this is what makes kumbhaka different from a common breath-holding. When lungs are wide, they don't press on the heart sac, allowing our heart to keep the same amplitude of contractions, without increasing the rhythm. This way we can understand the criteria of doing this exercise right, given in old books: **it makes the heart beat not faster, but slower.** If you neglect this particularity, this exercise, if done regularly, can influence very badly on our health.

Another important detail is banhas. Their role is the following: uddiana bandha provides the excessive pressure, intensifying blood circulation in lungs and raises Manipura energy to Anahata (especially important after Bhastrikas). Djalanadhara bandha in its turn prevents from the increasing pressure in the head (intracranial pressure). Indeed just try to release this bandha in the exercise and you'll feel a strong hydraulic hammer beat in the head. Muladhara bandha prevents the increasing of pressure in lower cavities of the body and the outflow of energy from lower chakras. From the above said we can understand the classical sequence of «taking» bandhas: djalanadhara — Muladhara — uddiana. It makes no sense to take them in any other order, for example, to do djalanadhara after uddiana, because the intracranial pressure is already raised. So the reverse release of bandhas is also understandable.

Djalanadhara bandha

---

[1] «Kumbhaka» means a pot, but it practically became a synonym of retaining at an inhalation.

Bhastrika (bellows)

Bhastrika is done in a similar manner as Kapalabhati, both in a more tough and amplitude way, with Manipura set-up. After the breathing cycle we do kumbhaka, lasting the time we were doing intensive breathing, i.e. at 20 breathing cycles kumbhaka must last for 10 seconds.

The inner criterion of doing Bhastrika right is the feeling of hot «fire» ball in the stomach. In kumbhaka this ball must rise to the heart zone.

Typical mistakes in doing Bhastrika

1. **Trying to breathe with the chest,** or worse, **«with the spine»** (i.e. bending and unbending the back). Bhastrika is so intensive, that breathing this way you can do some serious harm to your heart, as well as provoke some unpleasant feelings in the diaphragm.

2. **Tension in face, neck, sometimes arms and legs muscles** doing the breathing cycle. These strains are the demonstration of pathogenic arches and can be a field of further psychological work (see «Relaxation meditation»).

3. **Breaking breathing rhythm.** For beginners a classical rhythm of Bhastrika 3:1 can be difficult and, if you practice without awareness, you can easily switch to 1:1. This mistake can be corrected by training and gradual deliberate reducing of the exhalation time.

4. **Slower down the tempo.** People with weak Manipura can find it difficult to maintain the rhythm of 120 breathings per minute, so they try to slower it down. In this case Bhastrika doesn't produce the needed effect of heating Manipura, although it does no harm neither. This mistake can be corrected by training and the appropriate emotional state (slightly «wild») while doing this exercise.

Holding the breath after «Bhastrika» according to canons must be equal to duration of «Bhastrika» cycle, because, if you do about 2 breathes per second (like you should) and have done 20 counts, breath-hold is 10 seconds; if you did 40 breathings, the breath-hold is 20 seconds. This correlation favours balancing the content of carbonic acid and oxygen in the blood, but, if you need to stimulate yourself additionally, you can skip the breath-hold and do just the active part.

The energetic sense of breath-hold is to transfer the energy-ball from Manipura to Anahata and then to distribute it in the blood circulation. Once it's done, there is no need to hold the breath. Longer holds can be used by advanced practitioners to achieve subtler states.

A little comment on Pranayamas

86

Hatha yoga pradipika and yoga-tattva upanishada say that when a person does pranayamas, he can feel heat, vibration, shivering, humming and sweating. Physiologically it means that a sympathetic branch of ANS is activated. Energetically it indicates the moving energy. During yoga session vibrations can grow to body rocking. It should be avoided, because rocking the body we disperse the energy in it. You should try not to rock, but to «keep the moving» inside. The same with vibration: just being watched, it calms down — the channel is clarified.

When we practice yoga, no matter what the ambient temperature is, we start sweating. It means Manipura is activated, which internally makes some energies move fast. This sweat stays on the skin for a short time and in 5 minutes it is absorbed. It differs from the usual sweating by the smell. It is not advised to wash this sweat off, because you'll lose a lot of energy. You should wait till it gets absorbed or rub it into your skin. This sweat has a certain influence on people, because it contains pheromones, making us more magnetic to others.

Any uneven (including one-sided) appearance of sweat indicate some disbalance in chakras' work.

Finishing yoga session

Meditation on disactualisation (forming intention)

To practice yoga, if the practitioner does right the meditation on actualisation, he gathers the energy from all his occupations, which are done «on his energy». This condition is a must for a quality practice, but can lead to some curious consequences — proceedings, off which you take your energy, get suspended and just stop. That is why when you finish your yoga session, do a return meditation, remember all your nearest plans, goals and aims, people, you are responsible for, in this way giving back some energy to your proceedings, which are really worth it. This technique is called a «meditation on disactualisation» or a «forming of intention». A special mudra can help you to form your intention.

GENERAL RECOMMENDATIONS AS FOR THE METHODICS OF INDEPENDENT PRACTICE FOR BEGINNERS

Principles of independent practicing yoga

Doing yoga complex by yourself, you should pay attention to the following.

Entering and exiting every pose
A lot about it was said above.

Stable state of your consciousness while doing all the complex of asanas
Stable consciousness is controlled by the breath, which is a guiding thread long all the complex. Rhythmic breathing is done in one rhythm both in asanas and passing from one exercise to another. No breaks between asanas: to sit, to think, to recover your breath and continue — is unacceptable, because it makes you lose your energy and disperses your consciousness. You start a rhythmical breathing, which already warms up the body, then you come to doing asanas. **Entering and exiting asana should be done in the rhythm of our breath, not vice versa**. Every time your breath breaks up from the initial rhythm, there is a failure of consciousness. If such malfunctions become numerous, maybe, it indicates that during the complex you should do a meditation on actualisation.

If your breathing rhythm accelerates, after exiting the pose you should stabilise your breath. Normal breath means healthy heart.

Deep breath in asana intensifies its effect, creating an additional rhythmical strain of channels at inhalation. Such breath is called «a pump breath».

88

Sequence of exercises (running a little ahead)

A complex is built with groups of three postures in each group. Every group one by one should worked out the anterior-middle, the posterior-middle and the diagonal meridians. Every next group of three does the same thing, only more intensively.

Exercises with legs apart such as Bhujangasana, Pashimotanasana (konasana), and the pivoted Arthamatsiendrasana with everted legs help to cleanse side channels, located in anterior and posterior sides of the body, aside from the central line.

Bhujangasana with a «risen tail» — the bended knees, is a half-strengthening asana, which has a firming effect. Exercises for stretching work with the inner etheric; half-strengthening and strengthening — train the exterior etheric. **Stretching asanas cleanse the channels and move the energy in the etheric,** while strengthening asanas firm the energy and drive it into a certain chakra, helping to structure a firmer chakral field.

Groups of asanas are chosen to include all elements. For example, the warming-up provides Wood energy, stretching asanas — Water energy, strengthening postures — Earth energy, small pranayamas, if done right, is Fire energy, Akapalabhati and Kapalabhati is Air and Metal. All elements should be presented in a complex in the precise order. If you ignore a group of exercises, your elements will be imbalanced. For example, if you do everything, except the warm-up, in the long run you'll feel heaviness in your body, because there is a lack of Wood and Fire, while Earth and Water are trained a lot.

If not to do firming half-strengthening postures, you'll feel certain looseness, as if you wanted to set out and flow. Such asanas firm our body after stretching poses. Too much of strengthening poses on the contrary make us too firm. «Gym-holics», if they don't do the stretching, walk as if their body was constrained, because their channels are clogged. A wise trainer after weight-lifting exercises gives some stretching ones, otherwise the body loses grace and suppleness. What is the clogged channel physically? **As soon as we stop driving physical energy to a blocked channel, our tissues start transforming into fat,** because they lack energy. Either you lift weight from morning till dawn, or you put fat.

So, if you want to build your own complex, you'd better include a warming-up, some small pranayamas, at least three stretching asanas and some breathing exercises. Such complex first work out the joints, then small pranayamas work out the cardio-vascular system, then we activate our muscles — doing stretching postures, then we do some strengthening postures and finish with some breathwork. Sometimes we can swap strengthening and breathing exercises. If after yoga we have some unpleasant work to do, it's better to do breathing exercises before strengthening ones — to close the field. In other words, you firm your field, you feel good and it's easier to «put a wall»; otherwise, if you have breathed nicely and feel alright, you can easily let enter some bad energies and states you don't need at all. All this is important to take into account.

After aerobic exercises when doing mulabadha and other kriayas, it's advised to put some salt on tour tongue and to meditate at a dan-tian, until it starts pulsing. This has a juvenile effect.

> **WARNING!** I don't recommend for beginners to do *Sirshasana* (standing on the head posture), although surely it's very healthy and is one of the main poses in yoga. The problem is that, if you want Sirshasana make you good and no harm, you must have a healthy neck. And most of people today have neck osteochondrosis after years of stooping at the desk. If they do Sirshasana, their neck-bone can be jammed, as well as other problems can occur. That's why I strongly recommend doing Sirshasana from the second year of practice, when your neck is to some extent cured by simpler asanas.

Time for yoga

If you are a «night owl», you'd better not do yoga in the morning before your body wakes up, otherwise pressure changes can be significant. If you measure your BP right after you wake up, it is low, and then it eventually stabilises. Only then you can start practicing. If you are a morning lark, your blood pressure lowers before you go to sleep, so this is the bad time for practice.

Set-ups

All small pranayamas should be done with the Manipura set-up, i.e. after doing them you should be hot. Doing strengthening asanas, you should breathe rhythmically with Muladhara set-up — otherwise your channels can be blocked by some less subtle energy. In particular you should pay attention on how deep you breath is, i.e. when you inhale, **every breathing zone should be filled to the maximum.** I recommend doing especially strengthening asanas with Muladhara set-up.

Ajna set-up appears when you feel an exercise like an instrument of work with your body. For example, when we stretch our legs to sit into lotus — we do the stretching consciously, not automatically. So we are thinking how to stretch our leg so that it would be put into lotus. This is a conscious and sensible work. **When we practice yoga Ajna set-up should always be at the background.** Every exercise should be done not to sit the needed time in it, but to change yourself, clearly understanding that now with the help of asanas, pranayamas, mudras,

90

meditation and so on I'm working with my physical, etheric and astral planes. For example, you sit down to do a rhythmical breath. If some part of your body is not «breathed» enough, it should be breathed personally. After it is breathed, the warm feeling fills all your body. Listening to your body and using all known instruments to improve your state — that's what we call the Ajna set-up.

In Chinese tradition there is a meditation «just to sit». Just to sit and not be distracted, while behind you there is a man with a bamboo stick — walking and beating those who are distracted. It's not difficult to see when someone is distracted: his shoulders lift, his head and so on. In this case the role of the third eye is played by a man with a stick. It is not in our custom — everyone is his own third eye. Everyone decided for himself either he works in yoga or he is just spending time, because someone said it's good for health. It is good for health, if you know what you do, otherwise it's not good. It's not harmful, but with the same result you could sit and watch TV... Without consciousness the practice become religion.

How long should yoga session last

I think that a normal person can do yoga for not more than an hour a day. If you do it right, an hour is enough to fill you with energy. However there are three levels of training, three types of routines:

- to keep fit;
- to fill yourself with energy and to accomplish some life tasks;
- to change yourself.

The final criterion to define how long your session should be is filling yourself with the energy in the amount you need.

Natural way in practice

Yoga doesn't mean you have to force your body. You should come naturally to every practice. For example, some people ask: «What to do, if you don't withstand fasting?» Don't force it. Do some custom practice and once you'll have a **need** to cleanse your body. This feeling appears when you get more energy. This energy can't pass the blocked channels. Then you get a natural need to fast. If you force yourself, Ajna energy is used for your intestines.

The goal of yoga is not to do as many asanas as possible, but to bring harmony to your body. Doing practices, your body becomes healthier, more stretched, and some asanas become possible to do.

About lifestyle, or
How to start practicing

How to find time for practice

If someone decides as usual to practice «on Monday», «seriously», «some hours a day», he'll stand it 2-3 days, not more. The lifestyle should be changed gradually. Besides even if we do nothing, everyone is «busy» all day long. People have no free time, and what is worse, no free **energy**. That's why to start practicing, one should ask himself: what can I sacrifice? Let's start with 10 minutes, we all are very busy, but, if you think, you can always find some 10 minutes for something we can do without, like watching a soap opera or reading a newspaper or talking to your neighbour. **You must clearly understand, what you are sacrificing.** When you understand what you are sacrificing, time appears from some precise sources, not from nowhere; of course you should sacrifice things you don't need. If you decide to sleep less, when you body is already not sleeping enough, it will be «mad» at you. Sacrifice with something you don't need: a useless conversation, watching TV, drinking alcohol etc.

Attitude of others and attitude to others

When someone starts practicing yoga, he can be played two dirty tricks, concerning his closest surrounding. **The first trick** is to tell immediately everyone that you started practicing yoga. Dispersing the energy of your intention and the one for you spiritual development. «Gods like mystery», said in ancient time. Your practice will become efficient, if as less people as possible know about it. Demonstrating your belonging to yoga is a pride or shows that your chakras are loose (or both). What is worse, people with whom you share this news are rarely happy about your good starting. It's easier to be sceptic than altruist.

That is what **the second dirty trick** is about — people surrounding you don't accept your practice. It is inevitable not just because of our mentality and the wrong understanding of yoga by average person. People always start spiritual practices with the disapproval of others. This is a manifestation of **a principle of environmental resistance**, implying that the environment resists **a person going up**, growing. The same principle is true for social conditions: try to evaluate, how the attitude of others changes, when, for example, you are promoted; it is equally true for the personal growth. The environmental resistance should be overcome — it is the way the World tries you on your right to raise your status.

On the higher level the resistance can be even used to your good, as a source of personal growth. For instance when you do yoga, your family «comments» it, irritating you — try to figure out which energy you don't accept. Why? Which chakra is not integral? So much work to do.

People attract situations that hurt even more their not integral chakras (see the book «Theory and practice of psychological aikido»).

Can yoga be harmful?

Yes.

Practicing the wrong way a person can cause himself a big damage. The main and the most dangerous mistakes are:

1. Practicing wrong asanas and pranayamas. There was a lot said about defects and their consequences, but we'll remind you that regularly doing exercises the wrong way can lead to problems with the backbone (enforcing osteochondrosis) and with the cardio-vascular system (when you breathe wrong, you can strain your breath even worse).

2. A yoga complex built wrong, first of all uncompensated one, can lead to a significant changes in blood pressure (which you don't need), states of ANS and so on. Most often this happens when a person wants to do only the thing he does well and not those he really needs. The pride...

3. Traumas. Graduality — in everything.

REMEMBER, yoga is a way for wise people, it brooks no unthinking and fanaticism.

The contrary is also possible. A person does yoga for some time (or comes some times to a group session, which is more often) and starts believing that all his problems are caused by yoga. «At a sight of diseases a yogin who fears them, says: the cause of my illness is in yoga. This is the first obstacle in yoga», — writes «Yoga kundalini upanishada». It is obvious that yoga has nothing to do with this, it is just the way to take away the responsibility for your health. This is how the so-called defence mechanisms of our psyche act, but the discussion of them lies beyond the scope of this book.

PSYCHOLOGICAL WORK
IN ASANAS

*Physical moves don't help by themselves; concentration is neither
the only clue to success. The one who does both physical control
and concentration achieves a success and becomes immortal*

Isha Upanishada

Human psyche structure

As it was said above, asanas are not an end in itself of yoga, but an instrument of work with one's psyche. The clue to such work is a system of psychosomatic correspondence, i.e. the projection of psychological problems on certain parts of the body in the form of muscle contractions, strains, in extreme case of diseases in respective organs. However unlike our psyche, our physical body can be seen. Looking at it and analysing certain parameters, we come to conclusion about the general and current psychic state of a person. There is one more aspect: it's difficult to see and become aware of one's own psychological problems, because of the «defensive mechanisms» — special psychological obstacles, keeping a person from adequately evaluating his own state. A physical body can always be seen. It can't be hidden, so looking in the mirror, applying certain schemes, we can conclude about our real psychological state. And vice versa, activating certain parts of our body, working out our muscle contractions, we stimulate respective psychic functions and as a result — stimulate the development and opening of chakras.

From the esoteric point of view unconsciousness is a whole of experience that a soul received during all its existence, which influence a person in the form of needs and aspirations. Besides unconsciously we are keeping a pseudoexperience — memories about some situations, we didn't pass the right way, which as emotions and attachments continue influencing on our life, actually representing our Carma. Main characters of pseudoexperience are an emotional pomposity and its ability to «hitch up» people's attention. Indeed emotional reaction inhere animals, not people, but a layer-like structure of experience results in the fact that, if a person doesn't have his own experience of behaviour in some situation, he reacts according to his experience from previous levels; i.e. the violent reaction proves that he has no human's experience in similar situations and that he's accumulated a pseudoexperience of behaviour in these situations.

But from all the above said we mustn't conclude that people should suppress their emotions. On the contrary, suppressed emotions are a typical mistake done by people under the influence of superconscious directives. As a result, emotional energies excreted from the body don't come out of the aura, are not realized in a reaction, causing discomfort and stress in this situation and in future ones.

The fact that human consciousness «sticks» in the situations that we didn't work out, is also explained from the point of view of evolution, representing so to say an instinctive wish to «come back» and «replay» the situation, to get from it all needed experience, but, if this wish isn't actualised and is not consciously realised, what this chapter is dedicated to, such touching leads only to energy loss and its blocking in the past.

At first glance it may seem that the problem of cleansing our subconscious appeared with psychoanalysis and has nothing to do with the classical yoga, but to prove the contrary, we can just open «Yoga sutra Patanjali» and read its first lines.

«Yoga is liberation of Chitta from Vritti..»

What is that «vritti», preventing a Seeing person from «contemplating true images»? Psychologists perfectly know the effect of distorted perception under the influence of directives, emotional reactions and subconscious complexes. That is why there are enough reasons to claim that the process of «liberation of Chitta from Vritti» has a lot in common with what nowadays is called «the cleansing of consciousness».

Before speaking about precise methods of studying the subconsciousness, let's study the objects we can meet there.

1. Non-reacted situations.

2. Complexes.

3. Neuroses.

Non-reacted situations is a memory about situations, feelings and emotions that were not reacted as needed, i.e. for some reasons were suppressed and are hidden in the subconsciousness. In everyone's life such situations are numerous: starting from parents' inhibits like «don't you dare to laugh», «stop crying» (while a child needs it!), up to tragic life events we preferred to forget. **From the energy point of view non-reacted situations can be imagined as some clots of energy, stuck in**

the inner part of aura. When we relieve the non-reacted situations, we unblock these clots and release the energy, they contained.

Complexes are a form of reacting, realized or not, on an external stimulus (restimulator) well defined in advance. Such a stimulus can be a person, an object or an event. The reason why complexes appear, usually has to do with the existence of non-reacted situations. An object, which becomes a restimulator could be presented or related to such situation; facing it, a person partly remembers some unpleasant experience, related to this situation, energetically comes back to it. It becomes the vice circle: an object provokes again unpleasant feelings, proving even more the negative reaction on it.

Neuroses are a constantly presented psychological trauma, related to contradictions between person's wishes and his superconscious directives, which he can't destroy consciously.

The biggest damage from them is that they keep a certain part of our psychical energy «frozen», in addition to that a certain amount of energy is used by our inner censorship to keep these objects in our subconsciousness. Naturally it lower the energy potential of our consciousness. Besides occasional breakthroughs of unconscious complexes to the conscious level cause neuroses, symptomatically becoming apparent on our health.

The contaminated mind is especially dangerous for those, who do spiritual practices, because for such work you must change your worldview, which in its turn destroys our mechanism of censorship. Besides new directives can overlap the old ones, being in our unconsciousness, and cause additional inner conflicts. Without proper knowledge and critical attitude to one's experience a person risks to get some severe neuroses and even mental disorders. The most common is a situation where unconscious complexes of the practitioner are percept by his consciousness in a form of images and symbols, which he mistakenly interprets as a result of his «entering to astral plane» (of his Forces, God, opening channels and so on)...

All the said considered, I will emphasize again, that **a work over cleansing of the subconsciousness must precede more complicated spiritual practices.**

To work out the described physical constrains, we'll use certain meditations, which are given below.

Relaxation meditations

The principle of this meditation is based on the fact, we recall once more: human's psyche, his consciousness and subconsciousness are projected on his physical body, that's why all mental disorders have their physical embodiment. However unlike the subconsciousness, protected from the consciousness by the mechanism of censorship, the physical body is open to study and can be used as a bridge to enter the world of subconsciousness.

Usually the most of psychological problems lead to muscle contractions and to the distortion and inhibition of different reflexes. In our case muscle contractions will be used as a clue to introspection.

Basic technique of meditation

First step

Take a comfortable and stable position (at this stage it's better to lie down on your back). Try to relax in the following order: toes, feet, ankles, shanks, knees, hips, fingers, hands, wrists, clbows, forearms, shoulders, shoulder girdle, abdomens, back, neck, face, head. After ending this cycle of relaxation, come back to your physical body and let your thought pass through the same zones, thoroughly checking, if these muscles are really relaxed.

If you find a not relaxed muscle, try to relax it by the power of your will. If you fail, concentrate your consciousness on this muscle, focus on it, watching all appearing images and emotional states. You have found some non-reacted emotions. Try to understand and to feel the situation or the emotion you're seeing as deep as possible, but remaining calm as an inside observer. After this try again to relax this muscle. If you succeed, continue the examination of your body, repeating the cycle of eliciting with every not relaxed muscle. You can help yourself, asking questions like «what prevents me from relaxing» or «what emotion is blocking this muscle» and so on. If after understanding the situation you still can't relax the muscle, try one of the techniques given below or pass to the next muscle, consciously noting that you have an unsolved situation.

Pay special attention to those parts of your body that your mind tries to skip or «not to notice». It's the true sign that the most serious problems lie there and you see the defensive mechanism in action. Another most frequent defensive mechanism is a sudden ir- ritation, anger, a wish to stop the meditation immediately or at least to change the pose. Actualise this feeling and note, when it appeared — the corresponding part of your body also has big problems.

The first step is done when you succeeded in relaxing all muscles. Usually muscle contractions reflect rather shallow levels of our subcon- sciousness and contain emotions and feelings we have without realizing it in. That's why a good way to relieve them is to actualise the respec- tive feelings (see the previous chapter), which results in liberation of the energy of this feeling.

People usually have typical projections. For example, a tension in the knees is related to some hurry, extruded for the time of yoga ses- sion; in abdominal muscles — to a fear, in the neck — to some respon- sibilities not fulfilled or oppressed and so on.

> NOTE. During meditation after having achieved a deep relaxation, you can experience some abrupt convulsive movements of the body, scaring both practitioners and their teachers. 2-5 seconds after they are over, new muscle contractions appear. It's nothing bad, in this moment there is just an «open- ing» of a deeper still not cleansed level of subconsciousness and its projec- tion on the body. Start meditation from the beginning.

Second step

Face relaxation. This step is harder than the previous one, because up to 70% of emotions are projected on our face, moreover these emo- tions are much more defined than those controlled by our body. The principle of this meditation is the same: one by one relax your facial muscles, actualise your emotions, feelings and situations, hindering it. You should also understand that at each effort of your will your fore- head muscles strain, so at a certain point you should switch off your will. Approximate correlation is this: set jaw — anger, tension in upper part of cheeks — non-acceptance, in the throat — non-realised wishes to say something etc.

Third step

Viscera relaxation. You should pass to this step only after you mastered previous ones, because here you'll deal not with physical re- laxation, but with the feeling of relaxation of every internal, tracing sit- uations, hindering it. This meditation leads us to some even deeper lay- ers of subconsciousness and often opens some situations, which were the reasons of our physical diseases of respective organs.

> NOTE. Different parts of the same organ often correspond to different situ- ations.

Forth step

Bones relaxation can lead us to a subpersonal experience, that's why, if you are a beginner in meditation, you'd better skip it. Of course, in our bones there are no muscles, but there are etheric and astral planes, so some energy can also be stocked there, as well as the feeling of tension and relaxation.

Fifth step

Chakras and petals relaxation can be used to open respective chakras and to trace blocks.

Meditating in asana

If you reached the third step, try to complicate your meditation, doing it in one of asanas. In this case the weight is redistributed and some muscles you weren't even noticing while lying on the back, suddenly show themselves. Your goal is to learn to relax all muscles, not engaged in doing asana. For example, if you are in Bhujangasana, pay attention to your fingers. If you have problems with Anahata, they huddle up. In Pashimotanasana usually contract abdominal muscles and the groin and so on.

Meditation is considered mastered, if you can relax all idle muscles in any yoga posture.

If these techniques help you to study what is in your subconsciousness, or esoterically speaking, once you feel your astral body, find situations, bothering you, your non-reacted emotions and complexes, you can start its «cleansing». Methods of work with subconsciousness can be divided in two categories: *analytical* and *catharsis*.

Analytical methods are based on becoming aware of different subconscious objects, using their indirect demonstration (dreams, emotional stresses etc.). Realization liberates and restructures energy, «frozen» in deep (unconscious) layers of the aura, which makes it possible to use this energy. The oldest and, whatever paradoxical it may seem, the most worked over technique is the Buddhist vippasana[1]. Most of modern analytical methods go back to different schools of psychoanalysis.

Catharsis methods are based on the direct reacting of the feelings and emotions that bother us, with no need to realise them. Most of dynamic meditations are used as catharsis.

---

[1] See «Religious psychopractics in the history of culture».

Techniques of energetic «denouement» and reacting traumatising situations

Analytical techniques

Of course problem zones diagnostics by «relaxing meditation» is just the first step in spiritual work. The main goal is to achieve the energetic denouement of unfavourable emotional ties, or speaking psychologically, «cleansing of subconsciousness». Here are some meditative techniques you can use to do this work. These techniques can be done both in asanas (then you'll see that it works, if an unpleasant symptom disappears or, if a group of muscles that previously couldn't relax, finally does it) and independently from hatha yoga, but in both cases a well-done practice must reflect on your physical state.

«Replaying» the situation

This meditation can be a wonderful addition to the relaxing meditation and can be done either at the same time (situations are reacted at the moment they are found), or afterwards — in this case you act by a plan of work with these situations, that you do in advance.

Technique. Remember and actualise a life situation from your past that was physiologically traumatising. Putting yourself into the state of inside observer, mentally go back in the situation and try to replay it as precisely as possible. Identify with yourself in this situation and live it through from the beginning till the end with all emotions, observing yourself. Repeat several times until you feel a relief or unless you feel, that the situation doesn't bother you emotionally anymore. Sometimes those who practice this meditation fall into a short sleep — all this proves that the situation was replayed, i.e. there was an energetic disengagement. This meditation is successfully done together with the analytical one.

Letting go your feelings

At first glance this meditation reminds the relaxation meditation, but its priority isn't muscle symptoms, but actualised feelings. Its effect is based on the fact that all feelings, lived through and actualised, are liberated and left.

Technique. Actualise your feelings. Chose one of them and concentrate on it. Focusing consciousness on your physical body, trace, how this feeling projects on it in the form of muscle contractions, tensions etc. Keep quietly watching these physiological demonstrations of this feeling, until you see that contractions and the respective feeling become weaker and disappear.

Switch your attention to another important feeling and repeat the procedure.

Analytic meditation

The principle of its action is based on the destructive capacity of our analytical mind. This meditation aims to sweep off from our subconsciousness all bothering situations and parents' programs, we succeed to realise.

Technique. Remember a situation that bothers you or a situation, in which you think a program was imposed to you. By any analytical method analyse this situation and everyone who participated in it. It can be an analysis from the point of view of natural laws, given to work out this situation, of psychotypes and personal characteristics of its participants, of their blocks, their dynamics of behaviour and so on. The more complete and detailed your analysis is, the better this situation will be solved.

Playing with situation

Technique. Remember a situation traumatising you. Identify with the participant of it, keeping the state of «inside observer» Start changing the scenery of the situation, keeping its general core. For example, you can change the season, the weather, the environment, the look of people involved. You can try to change their size, making the most bothering images very small with a grotesque form, to change their voice (for example, make men talk with a little squeaky voices) and so on. This meditation is done well, if the anxious feeling for the situation diminishes.

What law is the situation for?

The following meditation is very effective, if done right.

Technique. Think of a traumatising situation. Realise the following: for which natural law did your Forces give you this situation? Characterise the behaviour you»ve chosen. (Note that the fact that this situation traumatises you guaranties that you»ve chosen it wrong). Build another line of behaviour according to the Natural Law you actualised.

The most common mistake in this meditation is to look for laws you already know, while in most cases situations are given to learn some new laws. Moreover, remember that laws rarely have a simple wording as «Don't do this or that». Most of laws have a more complicated and sophisticated form. Don't forget that a law is only a wording that regulates behaviour.

Letting go your thoughts
(great meditation of Tilopa)

This is one of catharsis meditations, done mentally. Its therapeutic effect is the cleansing of your subconsciousness from suppressed thoughts.

Technique. Sit comfortably and relax, let go your thoughts. Allow any thoughts come to your mind, staying like an inside observer to this without identifying yourself with your thoughts.

Soon when your common thoughts and the inner dialogue wear out from unconsciousness, on a conscious level would come some thoughts, that you may find wild, awkward, not yours etc. The most important in this meditation is not to resist them, just to observe them with no emotions and to trace them, accepting the fact that they are yours. Meditation should be stopped, when you feel a great discomfort or when you «lose yourself».

WARNING! Emotional people or those who have a weak Ajna-chakra shouldn't do this meditation.

All the above-described meditations, maybe except the meditation of Tilopa, are the simplest techniques for beginners. The scope of their usage is limited by situations, where there is only a personal trauma and no energetic connections with other people. Technologies of work with astral connections are the advanced level of yoga practice, which is beyond this book.

Catharsis techniques

From many catharsis techniques (see the book «Psychology of spiritual development»), the most suitable for asanas practice is the «astral breathwork».

Astral breathwork

Being in asanas some practitioners feel some pain and want to groan. The most often it happens when they are working with their anterior-middle channel, because in this part of the body accumulate emotions, which can be expressed. If such wish appears, it should be satisfied, i.e. groaned. It liberates suppressed energy and cleanses our astral body at the level of the respective chakra. If the reacting is done correctly, the muscle contractions may disappear at a physical level and feelings related to the movement of etheric energy become more intense.

102

STRENGTHENING POSTURES. TECHNIQUES OF FIRMING THE FIELD

Looseness and density of chakra

Let us briefly describe physical and psychological features, typical of looseness and rigidity of chakra.

By looseness of a chakra or of a field we understand such state of the field, when it can easily be breached, i.e. with the relatively weak energetic influence at the respective level appears «a hole» or an energy outflow. Too loose fields prevent energy from staying in chakra. Field's looseness is an unstable state: energy is present, but can't be kept. The etheric field is dense outside and looser inside.

At the behaviour level looseness is a state when a person hasn't yet worked out a certain «natural» law, but he hasn't got the situation on it either. Physically muscles at the level **of loose chakras are not developed enough or hypertrophied in relaxation.**

On the contrary **a state when a person can hardly emanate the respective chakra's energy is called rigidity.** Rigidity is a hypertrophied excessive density of energy. **Muscles in these zones are strained, stretching is harder.** The most often rigidity appears, where chakras are *blocked*. Note that, if chakra is rigid, it doesn't especially mean that it is weak. If a person has a rigid and weak chakra, he's very «lucky». At least he'll have no neuroses. If chakra is strong and rigid, a person constantly stays in the inherent contradiction, because the energy seeks to come out and finds no way out.

As other energy features, field's looseness and rigidity find their reflection on the physical body and on person's emotional state (astral plane).

Muladhara

The looseness of Muladhara at the behaviour level will show as a tendency to possess more property, than one can afford. **Muladhara's rigidity** is a state of constant squeezing of the pelvic floor. A person lives with a constantly locked mulabandha. It is quite frequent, because in European culture there is an excessive disgust for all processes that have to do with defecation, urination and so on. The psychotype of the person with rigid Muladhara is similar to the anally fixed type, customary in psychoanalysis.

A good example of an anally fixed type is Chekov's «man in a case». He dresses «for the case, if the weather gets colder». Every day is all the same: he goes to work, comes back home, on Sunday goes for a walk (from point A to a point B — all planned and fixed). This is the sign of rigid Muladhara, when a person is unable to digress from his customary schemes. Physically you may see Muladhara's rigidity as a strained pelvic floor and limited mobility of pelvis and hips. Usually such a person can hardly stretch his legs apart.

Svadhisthana

Loose Svadhisthana is easily diagnosed by an excessive mobility of the pelvis, which goes out of control. It is especially noticed when a person is standing. His pelvis always «falls out», often ahead. He moves his leg, and his pelvis falls out. It seems that his pelvis lives his own life. Sometimes you can notice that his underbelly (the zone between the navel and groin) is slightly falling out. At the behaviour level loose Svadhisthana leads to the fact that a person easily gets horny and can hardly get an orgasm — this is more typical for women. For men the sign of loose Svadhisthana is high excitability and quick ejaculation, caused by the incapacity to keep the energy. Easily getting drunk is also a sign of loose Svadhisthana.

Svadhisthana's rigidity is the incapacity to let out your sexual energy. This means a person can't admit that he has a desire, can't show this desire, sexually express himself etc. Physically it is a strain in the underbelly. Due to this the lower back arches and the pelvis goes slightly back. Funny, but a lot of models that are seen as an ideal of sexuality have the same posture. Such a person walks «like a duck» — his pelvis back. For a woman with a rigid Svadhisthana it's difficult to become excited, while a man is extremely shy.

Manipura

A loose Manipura results in a behaviour called being bully. A person has a tendency to take more than he can bear. A person with a loose Manipura typically has a «soft belly».

Note that men get looser Manipura after they get married. He has already reached something, has a family, a quite good financial state, he doesn't feel like fighting anymore, he has some stability, there are people, on whom he can count... A person is «realized»: partly gave his Manipura to a company, partly — to his wife, partly — somewhere else. Everything seems alright, but any stressful situation breaks him down, because his Manipura is delegated. In this case appears the belly. Women can also have it, although men have it more marked.

A rigid Manipura is a state with the constantly strained abdominal muscles. Normally this state doesn't last long, because it easily ends with the stomach ulcer. A person constantly stays in the state of strongest not expressed inner aggression — «a boiling copper of rage». The most often this aggression is transformed into autoaggressiveness, causing ulcer.

Anahata

For men **a loose Anahata** is difficult to diagnose, because they have not much to see. For women it's more obvious. Usually when her Anahata gets looser, her breasts grow flabby. Until a young girl or a woman is living with her own bright emotions, being a source of them herself, her breasts «stand high». As soon as emotions become weaker, a woman starts «following» the emotional sphere of others, her breasts grow and start hanging. Emotional looseness of Anahata is expressed in the fact that a person is easily influenced even by slightest emotions. The typical person with loose Anahata watches a soap opera and sobs, when a bad guy tortures an innocent pure heroine.

Rigid Anahata can be easily seen. In our culture it is quite often because of our upbringing. The easiest way to diagnose it, is by problems with breathing (incapacity to breathe with the chest). Psychologically Anahata's rigidity is the incapacity to express your feelings. A person can have feelings, but he fails to express them, to let go. Often he doesn't even know that he has these feelings. He feels not quite comfortably, but he can't define his state more precisely and understandably. It's a problem of our culture: «do I love or don't I love, do I love or do I hate — I don't know». If feelings are blocked, but the chakra is strong, they still try to come out somehow, «tearing a person apart», and his chakra gets breached.

Vishuddha

A loose Vishuddha is seen by the fuzziness of speech and by many fillers in it. If a person speaks a lot, but it's difficult to understand what he wants, his Vishuddha is strong, but loose. Talkativeness is a sign of loose Vishuddha.

Especially, if a person gives information, he'd better kept for himself.

A rigid Vishuddha is diagnosed by a constant hypertrophied strain in the neck. Sometimes these muscles are so strained, that the person starts «playing» with them, because muscles can't stay in tension for a long time and must be released. That's why this tension is not realized at all.

A person with rigid Vishuddha has something to say, but has no right to do it. Another alternative of rigidity is the rigid neck. In this case it is a sign of hyper responsibility, when a person can't say «no». He takes upon himself too much, and it becomes a burden, pressing him to the ground, ultimately causing neck osteochondrosis.

Ajna

A loose Ajna is an attribute of a person with the superficial worldview. As soon as he sees a new idea, he goes for it, especially, if it is well presented: «We drink «Herbalife»?» He'll sincerely persuade you to drink «Herbalife». Then another idea — we should give ourselves an enema — let's give enemas. He's jumping from one idea to another without making a critical analysis of each concept to synthesize it in his worldview, instead he's jumping from one to another — like on the waves. Those ideas can even be contradictory. Unfortunately you cannot diagnose loose Ajna by the expression of the forehead.

A rigid Ajna is seen in constant wrinkling of the forehead, in the conviction that you must always be thinking, or in the hypertrophied tension in the eyes. Ajna's rigidity often doesn't relate to it directly, but appears after blocking tears for a long time. A child is forbidden to cry, then he prohibits himself to express his emotions through the eyes. A constant tension appears in periocular muscles, emotional tension accumulates. At the behaviour level the Ajna's rigidity is showed in the incapacity to accept other points of view and to enlarge one's worldview.

The sign of looseness for every chakra is that it can be easily breached. For example, a slightest emotional influence by Anahata — you walk and see a dead cat — tortures you, because you easily take this state on yourself. It's a sign of loose Anahata.

106

Strengthening asanas

Strengthening asanas fix the looseness of our etheric field, dense it. Unlike stretching and pivoting postures, their effect is based on attracting energy to the most strained zone of muscles. **Physiologically this influence is noticed by the muscle vibration in the involved zone**. If there is no vibration, the pose is done incorrectly. **In strengthening (tightening) poses one should stay quiet long, overcoming the resistance**. If you do these poses till «the slightest discomfort», it gives no effect. The unwillingness to withstand difficulties, to exert oneself and to feel discomfort — these are astral signs of a loose field; and vice versa, tightening etheric field stimulates these qualities.

In strengthening postures you should pay attention to your breath, which has a tendency to break. **Indeed, uncontrolled emotions mean the field is loose**. Our consciousness is the mirror of our breath. If the breath is broken, the flow of consciousness is broken as well.

In case of muscular overstrain or excessive fatigue after doing force postures adverse effects can be relieved by doing Bhastrika.

Tightening Manipura field

Parvatasana
Forward set (mountain pose)

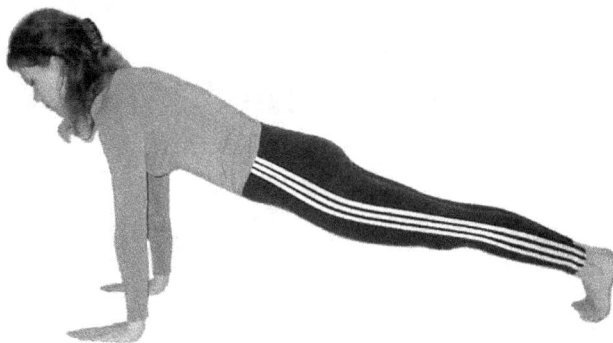

This pose stabilizes and tightens the etheric of anterior Manipura.

Technique. Take a push-up pose, on your hands or on your wrists under you shoulders, hands parallel. Shoulder blades aren't risen, pelvis isn't falling down. Stand in this position until you feel vibration in you abdominal muscles. Sometimes there is also a vibration around kidneys. The effect from asana can be intensified by mantra «houm».

Criteria of doing right. Vibration in abdominal muscles.

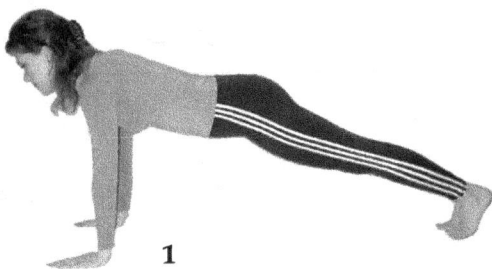

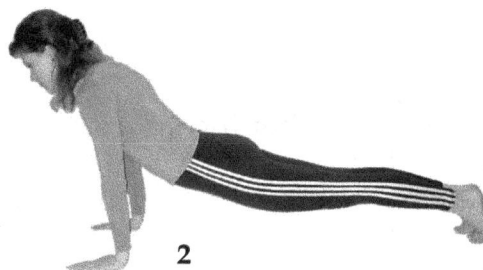

Mistakes in doing parvatasana

1 — curving the back with shoulder blades and pelvis — typical for people with rigid Svadhisthana; 2 — sagging typical for people with loose Manipura. In both cases Manipura isn't tightened.

Parvatanasana
Backward set (mountain pose)

This asana tightens the etheric field of anterior Manipura.

Technique. The same as in the previous pose, only face up.

Criteria of doing right. Vibration in the lower back.

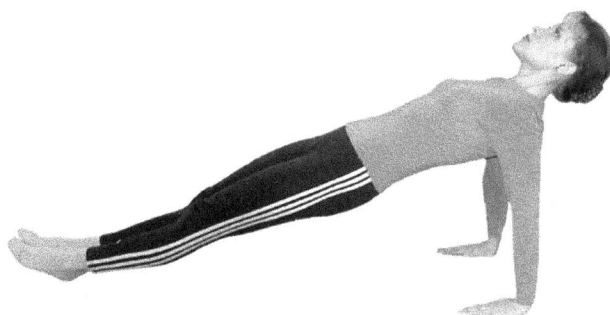

Tightening Svadhisthana field

Kandharasana
Set on shoulders (shoulder pose)

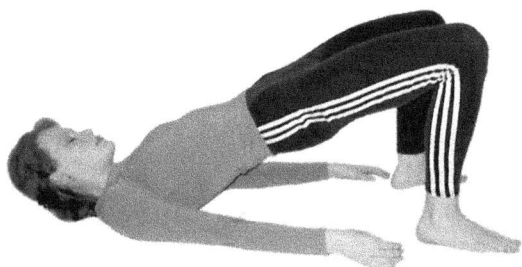

Technique. Stand on your shoulders. Lie on your back, bend your knees and put your feet close to your hands. You can grasp them. Rest upon your nape and your shoulders.

Criteria of doing right. Vibration in the underbelly and in anterior hips.

Arthasalabhasana (half-locust pose)

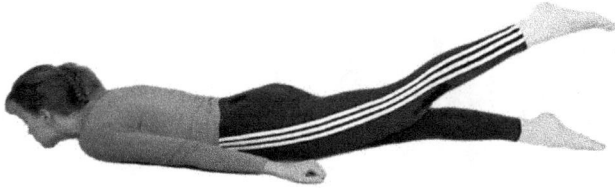

Starting position. Lie on the floor face down. Arms long your body.

Technique. Raise one leg, not bending the knee and not taking your pelvis off the floor.

Criteria of doing right. Vibration in the zone of kidneys. The most typical mistake in this exercise is to raise the pelvis from the floor and to raise the leg by pivoting the back. Then the needed effect (tightening of the field and vibration) isn't achieved.

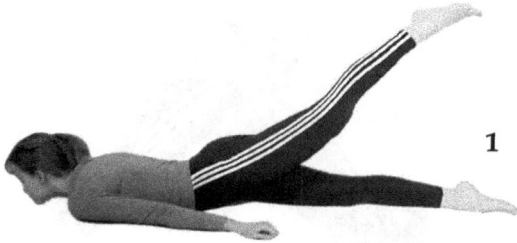 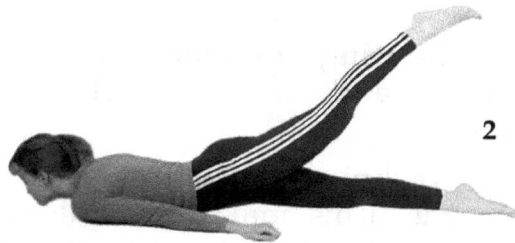

Mistakes in doing Arthasalabhasana

1 — the pelvis is raised off the floor (the pose looks more impressive, but doesn't tighten the field); 2 — the same plus the pose is done by pivoting the backbone. Can cause traumas to a weak or ill low back.

Salabhasana (locust pose)

The same as the previous one, but raising both legs. The effect is similar, but stronger.

Dhanurasana without hands (bow pose)

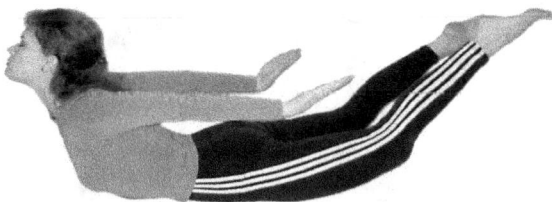

Starting position. Lying on the belly, hands long the body.

Technique. Raise straight hands long the body, raise and keep legs up, feet together.

Urdhvadhanur asana
(inverted bow pose)

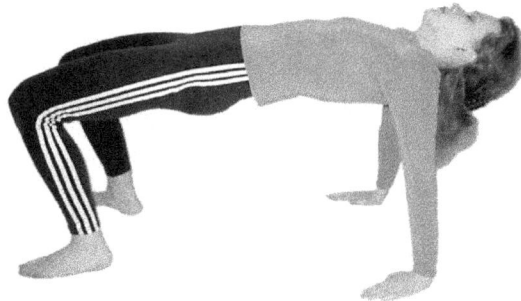

Cat pose

Starting position. Lie face down, hands at the level of the chest.

Technique. Lift your pelvis so that the arms make one line with the back. The back must be straight. The bending is done only by the pelvis. Don't bend your knees. Heels, if possible should stand on the ground.

Criteria of doing right. Vibration in lower part of stomach.

Mistakes in doing cat pose
Round lower back. Svadhisthana field wouldn't tighten, because the energy will accumulate in the belly.

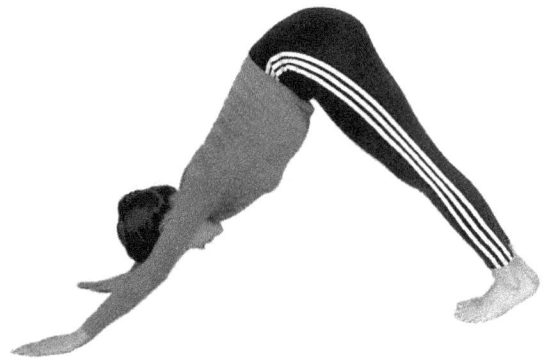

Advanced level of the exercise

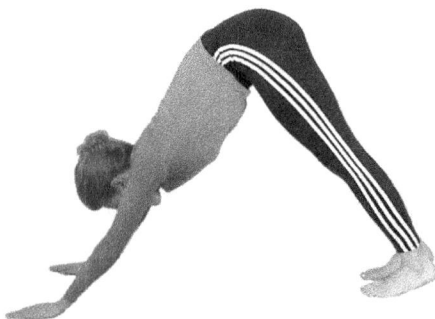

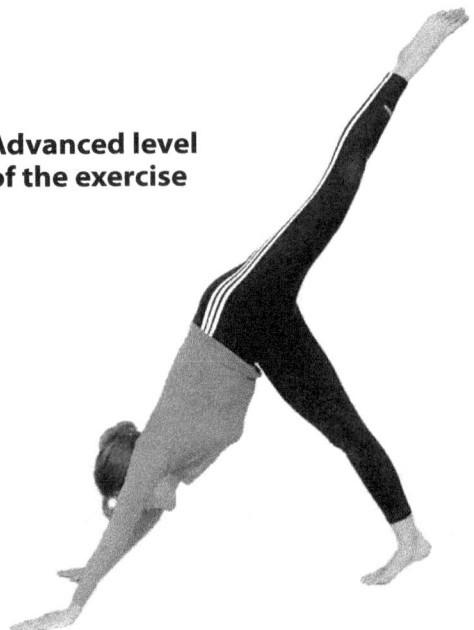

110

Navasa (boat pose)

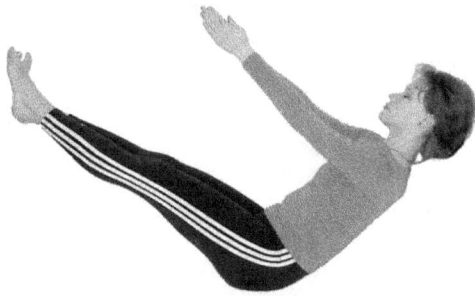

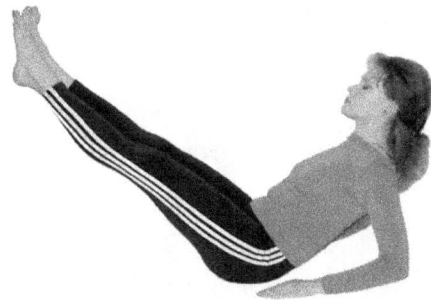

Navasana   **Simplified version**

Firabhadrasana (swallow pose)

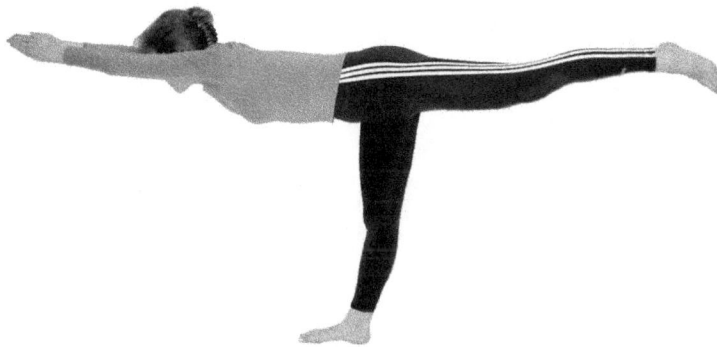

Tightening Muladhara field

Kukutasana (cock pose)

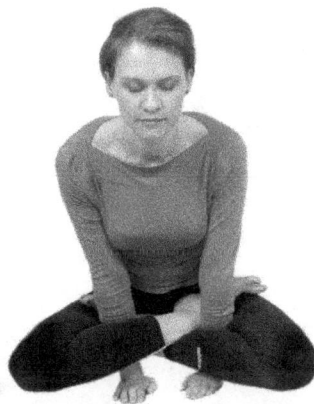

Controlled splits

Legs apart in splits, thigh muscles fixing it. The tension in inner thighs muscles stabilises the looseness of Muladhara. The most important in this pose is not to move the pelvis.

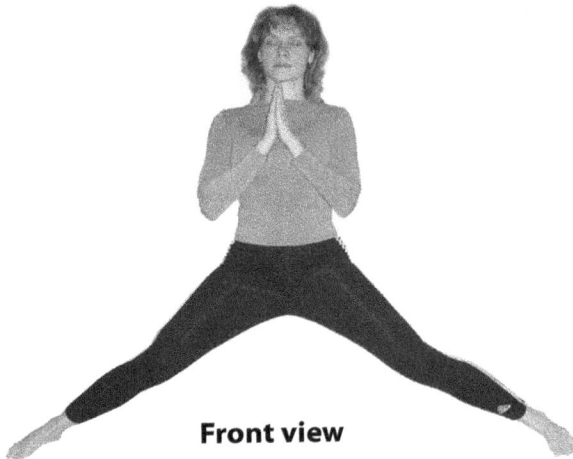

Front view

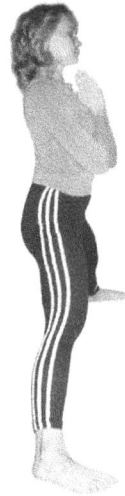

Mistakes in doing splits
The pelvis is moved back

Uttkatasana (strong pose)

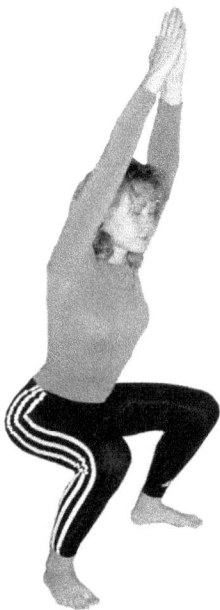

Uttkatasana

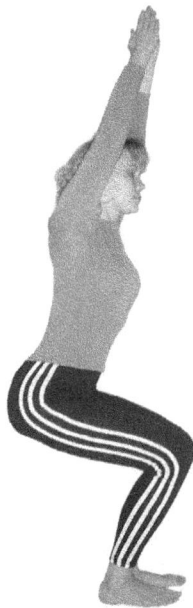

Uttkatasana with feet together

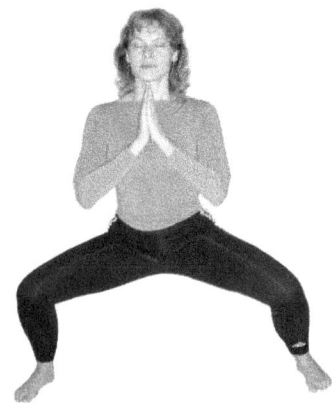

Simplified version
Horseman pose in qigong

Tightening side zones

Santolanasana (balancing pose)

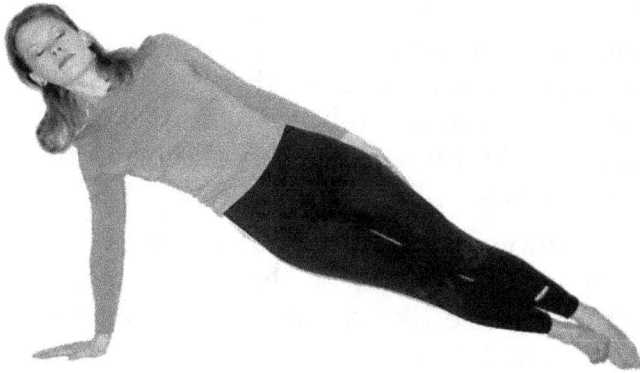

Uthita parsfaconasana
(stretched right angle pose)

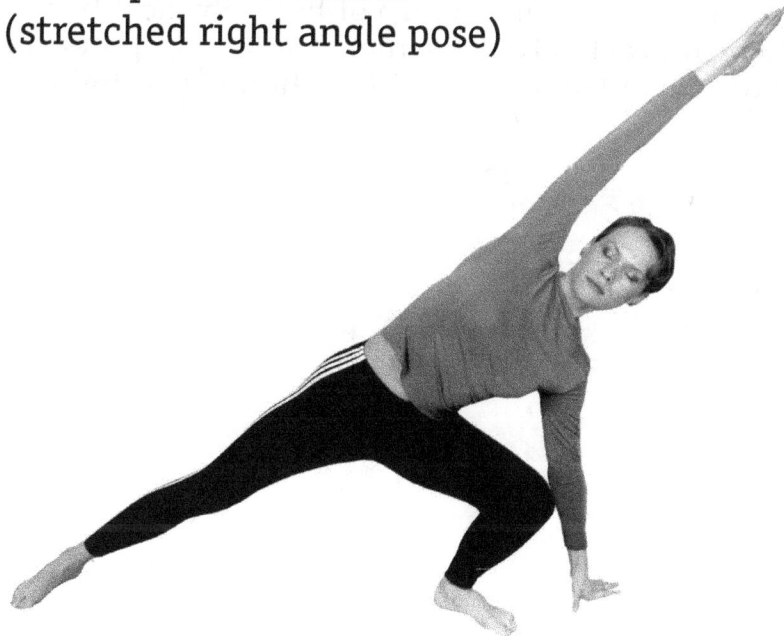

Strengthening poses
in yoga complex

Strengthening poses is an important part of yoga practice, even if the practitioner has no looseness in his chakras. Doing the stretching we cleanse our channels, move energy in them, our etheric starts «swelling». Evidently we become more energetic, but then the energy is easier to lose. To make sure it doesn't happen, stretching asanas should be compensated by tightening postures, i.e. by asanas, which condense our etheric, tightening it in respective zones.

Tightening poses should always be compensated with stretching poses, in a very proportional way. If you do only tightening poses, your etheric will be rigid, i.e. you'll move like a soldier. If you do only stretching, you'll become too loose, like a «dust in the wind», which is also bad, especially for the social life.

Yoga always means a good balance of flexibility and density, largeness and building-up of both physical body and physiological state (which is actually the same). Tightening poses are well done with tightening meditations, i.e. with techniques to tighten the astral field.

ADVANCED EXERCISES AND THEIR ENERGY INFLUENCE

Modifications and variations of main asanas

As it was said above, if practiced regularly, one can get used to yoga postures. Asanas and pranayamas, which were influencing greatly the state, causing significant feeling of the energy movement, become usual and stop making the same effect. Here is the mechanism of this adaptation.

1. Our body accustoms to the same workout. Practicing asanas, we enlarge the capacity of our body — the physical and the energy one. To neutralise this adaptation we use advanced variations of asanas.

2. «Unfreezing» of the most significant zones of the «blocked» energy, which used to be the source of strong sensations. To avoid this adaptation one should include into his practice some techniques to get energy from outside (see «Techniques of work with energy»).

3. Psychological adaptation to new sensations, which makes the actualisation to practice exercises less stable. Your attention and energy are dispersed. To avoid this adaptation you should use more regularly the meditation on actualisation while doing exercises.

To keep yoga practice effective we can use more difficult exercises. These advanced asanas can be useful for people with naturally high flexibility. The analysis of these exercises shows, that by their work, and by their energy effect and sensations, **these asanas are similar to the basic ones, described in the previous chapter**.

The contrary is also true: the need to practice advanced asanas comes only after the reserve of basic ones is over. Otherwise more complicated asanas will only exhaust inside reserve of the body. As it is said in «Shvetashvara upanishada»: «If you cannot master all asanas, master just one, but reach the total comfort in it».

So let's take a look at some advanced yoga postures, which can be used after the total mastering of basic exercises, taking into account the inner criteria of mastering.

Bhujangasana
and its variations

**Bhujangasana with
an advanced bending,
resting on hands**

(2nd variation of Bhujangasana)

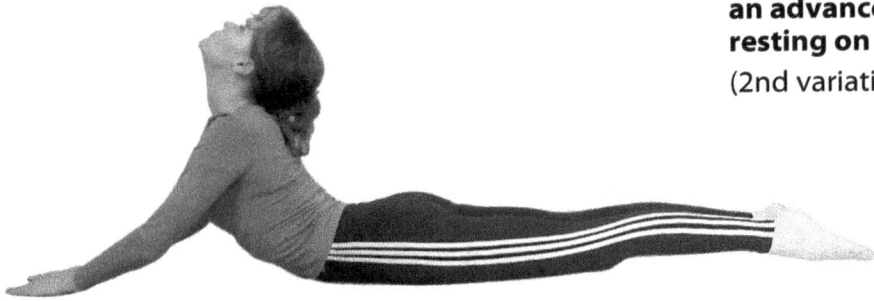

**Bhujangasana
legs apart**

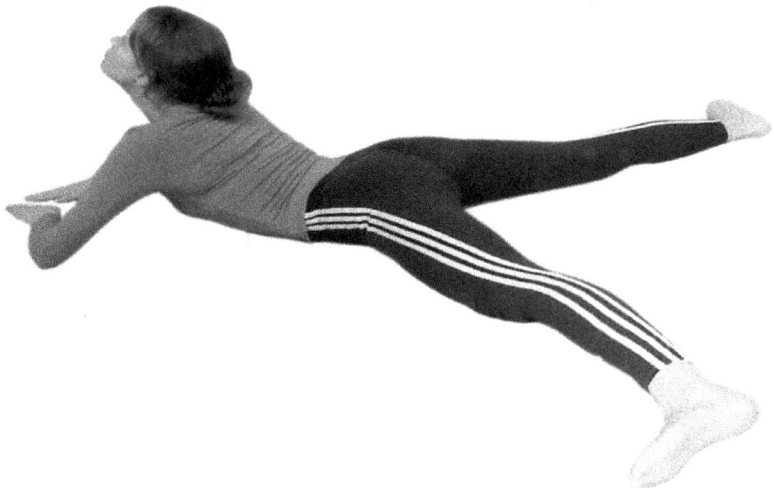

**Bhujangasana legs
bended in the knees**

(3nd variation
of Bhujangasana)

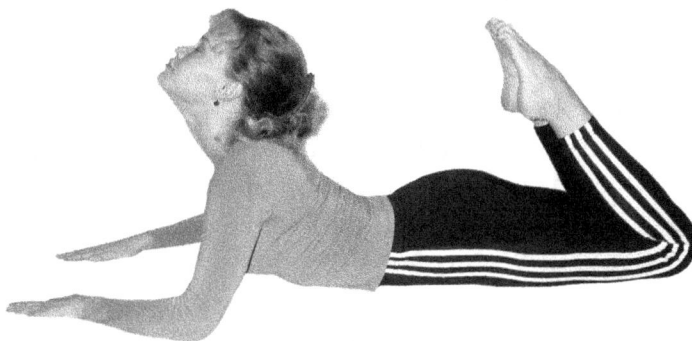

The general feature of postures with legs apart is that they drive the energy not by the anterior-middle channel, but by the meridians of the anterior and posterior parts of the body, on the sides from the middle channel.

Asanas
similar to Bhujangasana

These asanas are done to stretch the anterior-middle meridian. Like in Bhujangasana, these poses should be entered from the top down, arching the spine vertebra after vertebra. If done correctly, these asanas make the energy move and cause the feeling of heat moving up the spine.

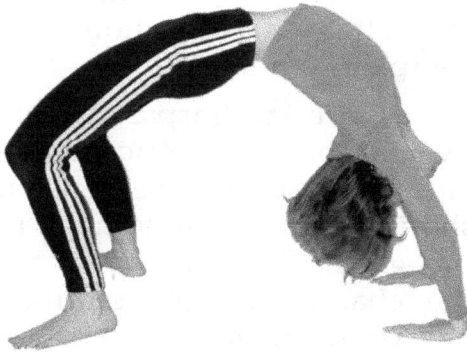

**Chakrasana
(wheel pose)**

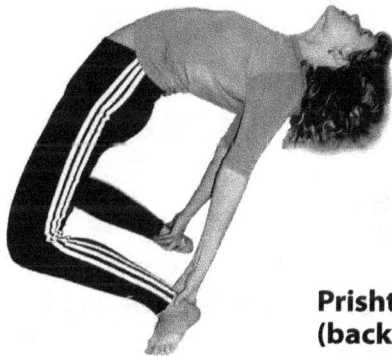

**Kapaliasana
(head stand
resting on the
forehead)**

In this pose there is a natural stretching of the anterior-middle channel

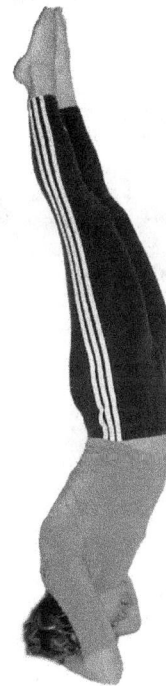

**Prishthasana
(back pose)**

Sarpasana
and its variations

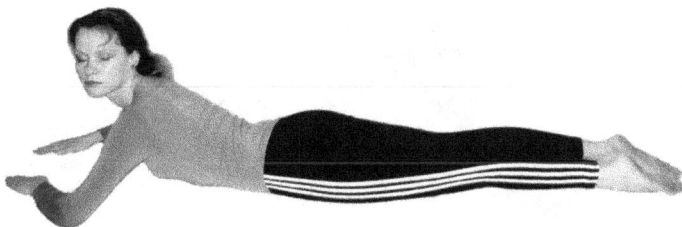

Sarpasana (snake pose)

Sarpasana is an exercise joining the effect of both Bhujangasana and pivoting postures. It is entered from Bhujangasana by turning the head followed by shoulders vertebra per vertebra, from the top down.

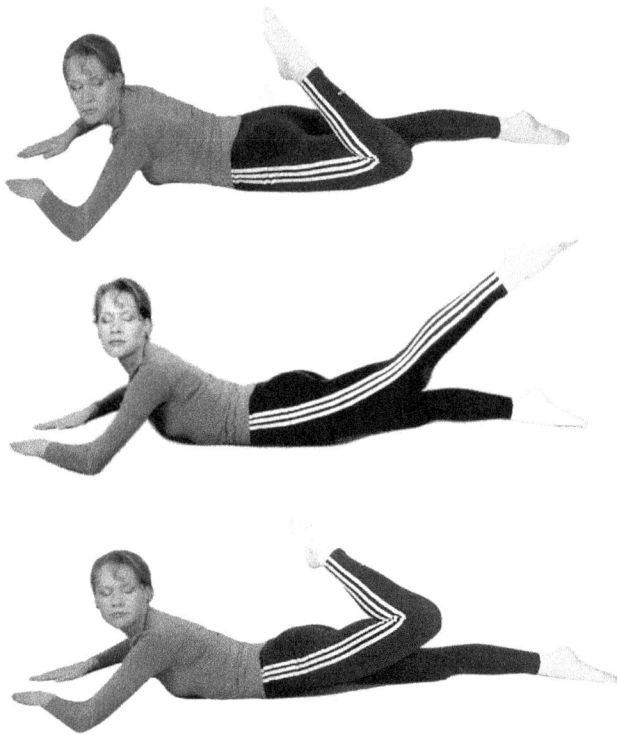

Sarpasana. Advanced variations. Various sarpasanas activate different back meridians. The more complicated it is, the closer to the spine energy moves.

Particularities of performing. In sarpasana one half of the body should be totally strained, and another — completely relaxed.

Criteria. Sarpasana activates non-symmetric meridians, that's why the tension should go from a temple to the groin. The heat goes up the channel on the strained half of the back.

Asanas similar to Pashimattanasana

Konasana (angle pose)

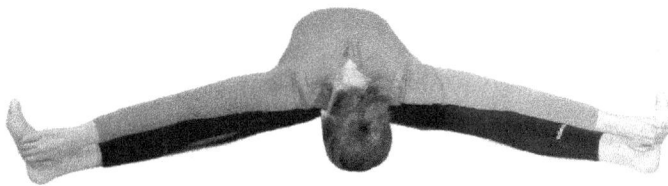

It's recommended for practitioners with the high flexibility of their lower back, who can't get the energy effect from Pashimottanasana.

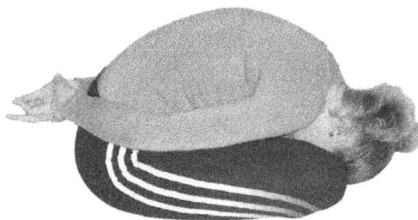

Yoga mudra

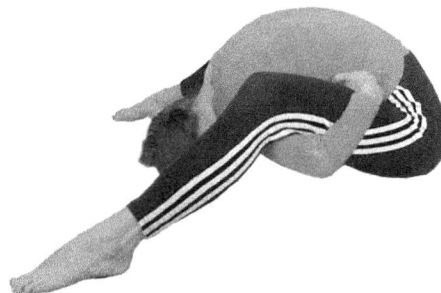

Kurmasana (tortoise pose)
For even more flexible people

118

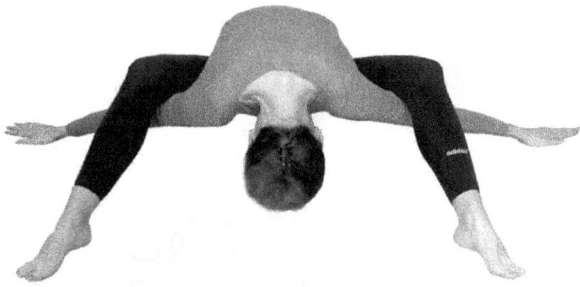

Kurmasana (tortoise pose)
Simplified version

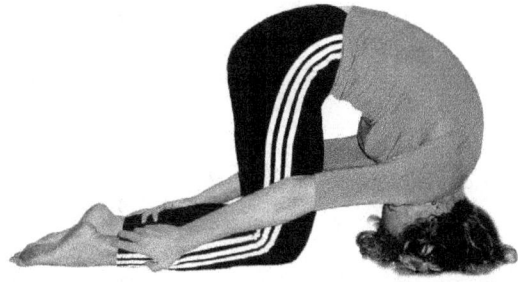

Pranamasana (bow pose)

Marichasana (Marichi pose)
The starting position for this
pose is Pashimottanasana

**Inside and outside
criteria** of doing these
asanas right are the same
as for Pashimottanasana.

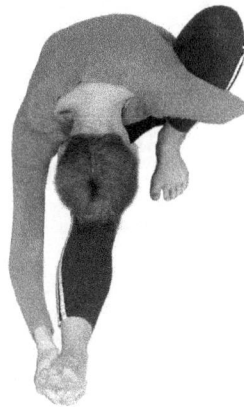

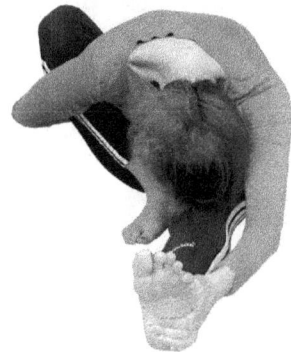

Arthamatsiendrasana
and its variations

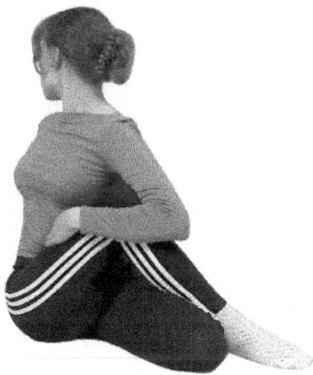

The pose is aimed to activate
the channels on the side of the
middle channel

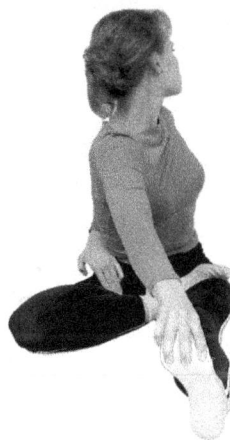

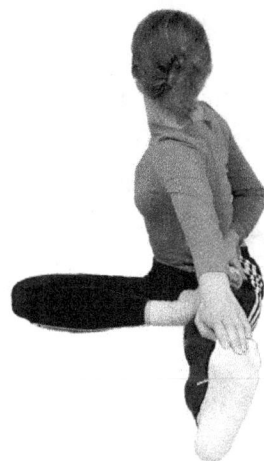

Poses activate meridians of the posterior
part of the stretched leg

Asanas
similar to Padahastasana

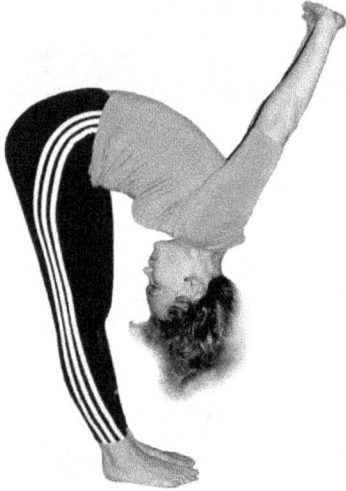

Dvikonasana
(double angle pose)
Intensifies the influence
on the posterior middle
channel

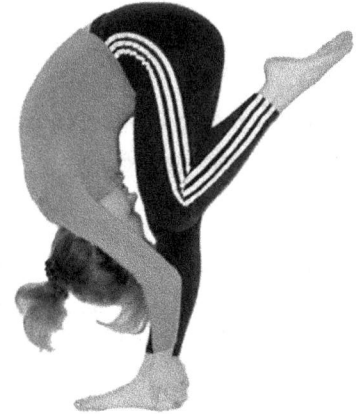

Padahastasana with
a bended knee
Intensifies the influence
on the channels of the
bearing leg

Trikonasana
and its variations

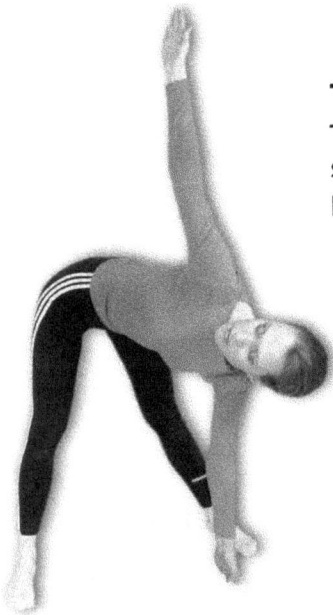

Trikonasana. First variation
The hand is put near the
same foot. The asymmetry of
poses is done by the pelvis

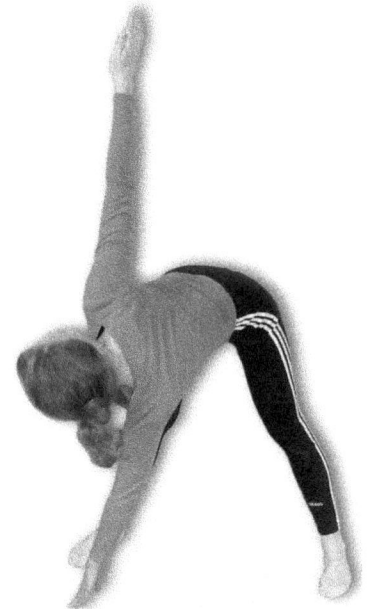

Trikonasana.
Second variation
The hand is placed near
the opposite foot

The inside criteria of doing these variations of Trikonasana correctly are the same as for the basic pose, described above. The only difference is that the strain is done only by one leg (to which the bending
is done).

120

Asanas
similar to Halasana

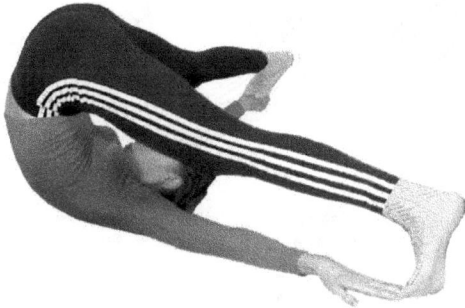

**Urthvakonasana
(inverted angle pose)**

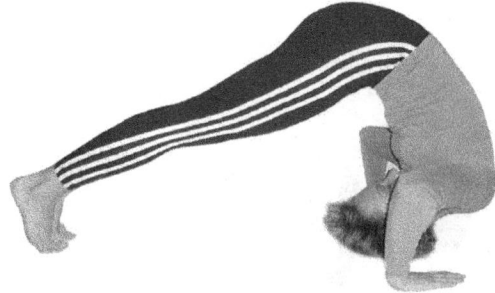

**Chakrasana kriya
(moving wheel pose)**

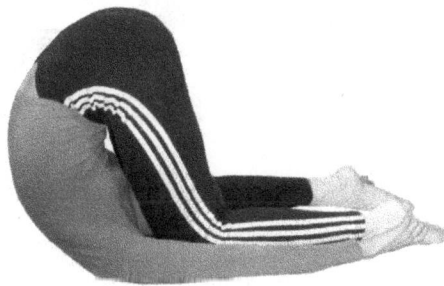

**Karnapidasana
(knees near ears pose)**

«Artha»-asanas
(asymmetric postures,
influencing side
meridians)

Asymmetric poses activate peripheral channels (lying aside from the central line and parallel to anterior and posterior middle meridians). Often the names of these poses have a prefix «artha-», meaning «half». It doesn't mean that «half-poses» are easier to perform than their complete versions. They just have a specific influence on **one half** of the body.

Athabhujangasana

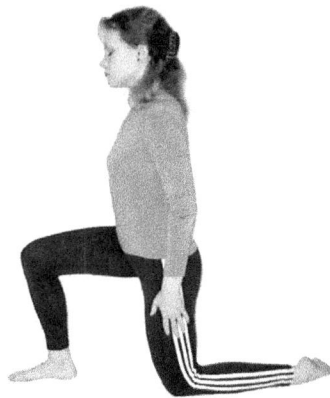

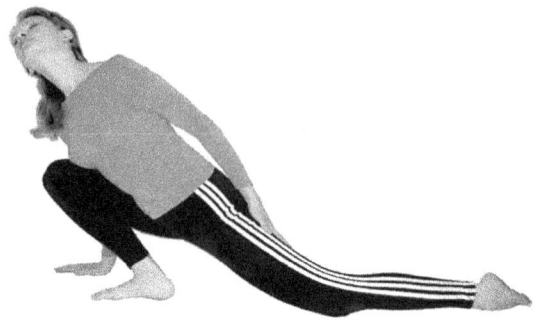

**Phases of entering
Athabhujangasana**

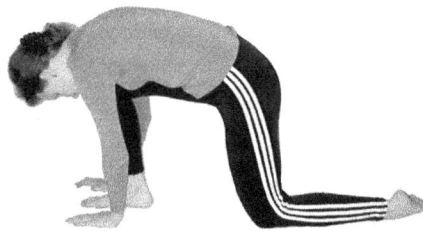

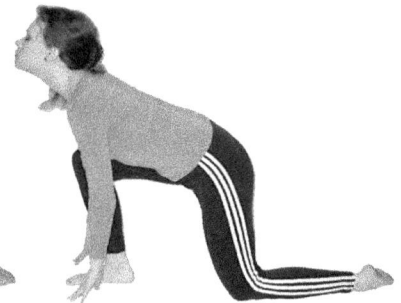

Arthanurasana

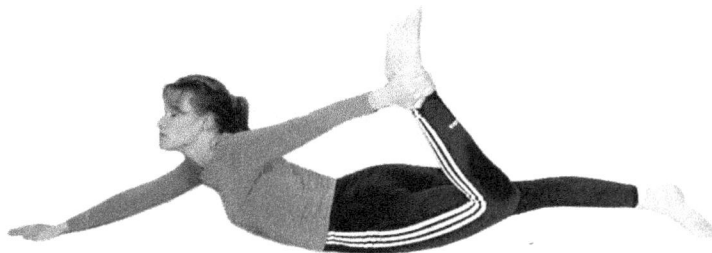

Arthaushtrasana

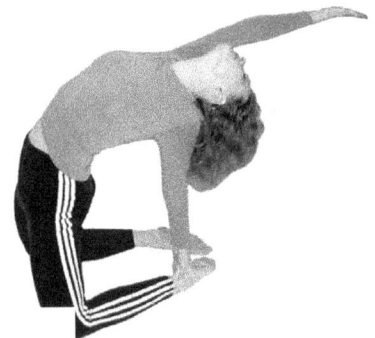

Virasana (hero pose)

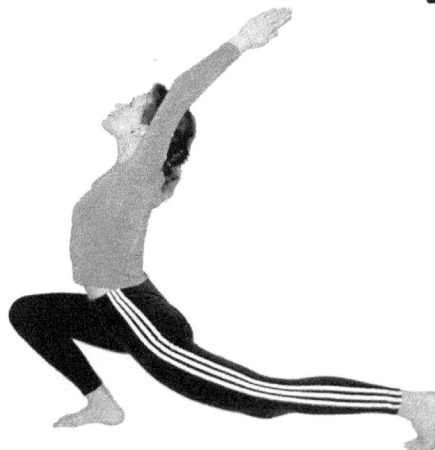

Arthapashimottanasana and its variations

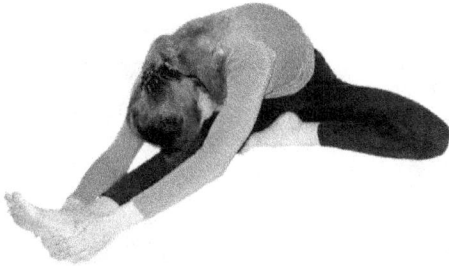

Djanu-sirsasana (head to knee pose). First variation

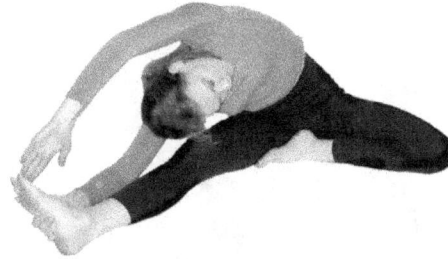

Djanu-sirsasana (head to knee pose). Second variation

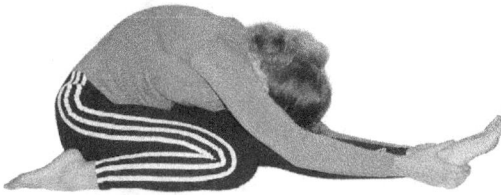

Triang mukhapada Pashimottanasana

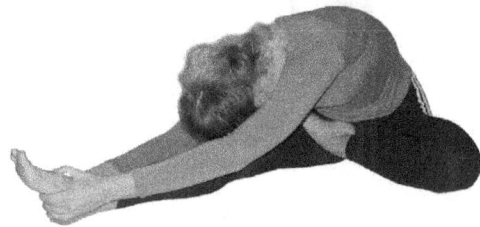

Athabaddha Padmapashimottanasana

Arthapadahastasana and its variations

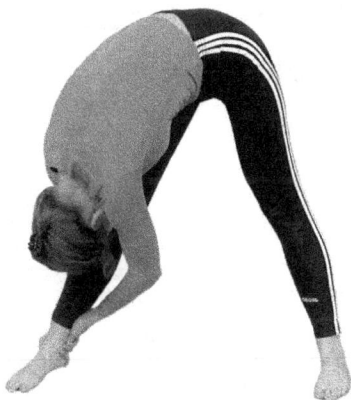

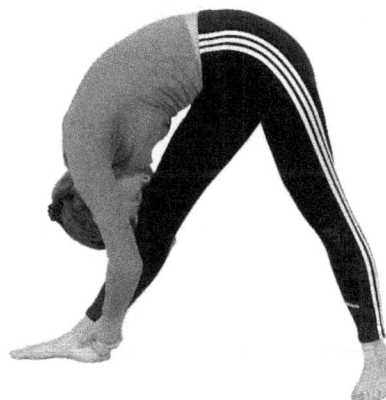

Parshvatonasana (stretching to Bhujangasana pose)

NOTE. Despite the formal resemblance, these poses activate completely different channels.

Sivanatarajasana
(Siva-Nataraja pose)

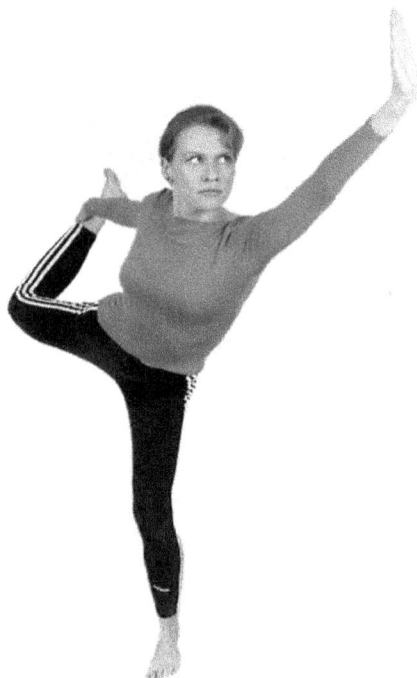

Tadasana

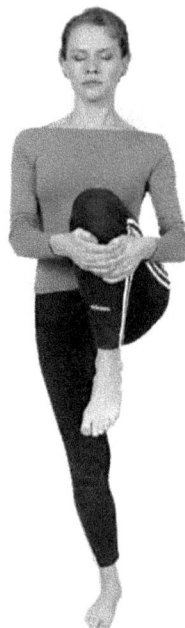

Mistakes in doing Tadasana

Bearing-out the hip closes the side meridian

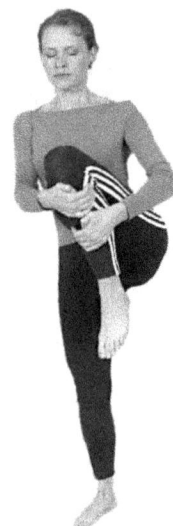

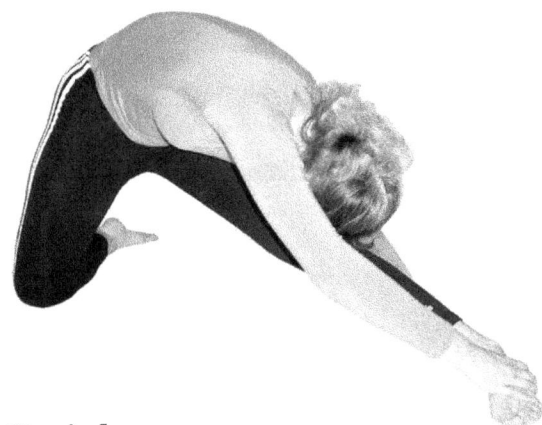

Parsva Halasana
(Halasana with a turn)

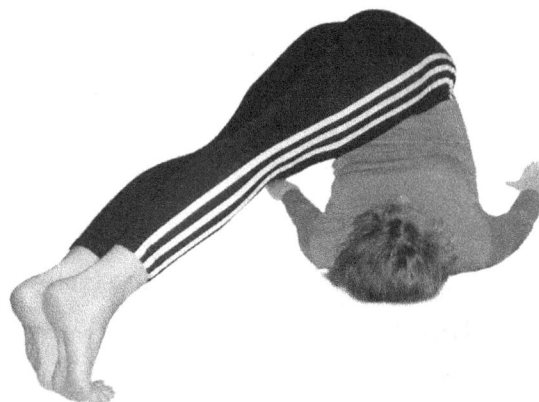

Parighasana
(crossbar pose)

124

Inverted poses

Viparita karani
(back movement)

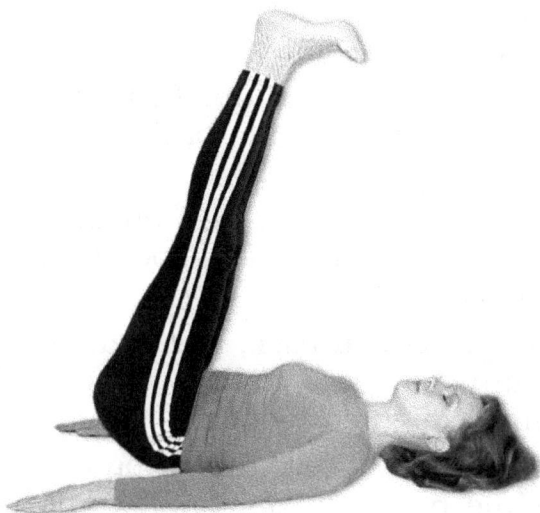

Viparita karani is a very difficult pose. To do it correctly, one must have a flexible pelvis zone. Actually it is a half-inverted, half-strengthening pose.

Starting position. Lying on the back.

Technique. Lift your feet in the way that your toes reach the level of your nose, pelvis isn't taken off the floor. The back must be straight, legs are also straight at a angle of approximately 70° at your body, the coccyx lying on the floor, no «arching» in the back. It's a half-inverted strengthening pose.

Effect and action. This pose tightens the field in the anterior part of Svadhisthana, pushing the energy up the anterior-middle channel. This effect is achieved, only if the back is perfectly straight and horizontal. Viparita karani does the same effect on women as nauli on men — makes the sexual energy (its etheric constituent) rise. It can be useful as a way of curing frustration, caused by sexual dissatisfaction.

Mistakes in doing viparita karani.
The back and the pelvis are taken off the floor

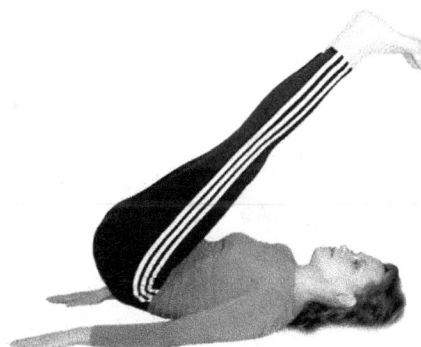

125

Sirshasana
(standing on the head)

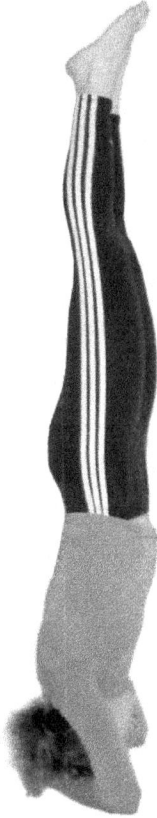

Sirshasana is one of the most important postures in yoga, rejuvenating all the body. However it should be practiced only after all the problems with neck osteochondrosis are cured (the best practice for it are sarpasana and pivoting poses), because otherwise it can provoke vertebra jamming.

Sirshasana isn't always easy to do. To master it one shouldn't be afraid to fall on the back, and for this it's helpful to practice somersaults.

Starting position. In vadjrasana rest on the top of the head, put your hands on the nape (fingers overlap, but aren't crossed).

Technique. Straighten you back, feet coming to your head, unbending your knees. Take your feet off the floor and carefully straighten them.

Effect and action. Sirshasana redistributes the blood in cavities of the body and makes it come to the head, if the neck isn't jammed in the exercise. The feeling of energy «coming» into the head is the sign that asana can be finished. Besides in this posture the muscles, responsible for balance are also energized. Which group of them — depends on the bearing area, i.e. on how hands are placed (for more details see chapter «Asanas boosters»).

Phases of entering Sirshasana

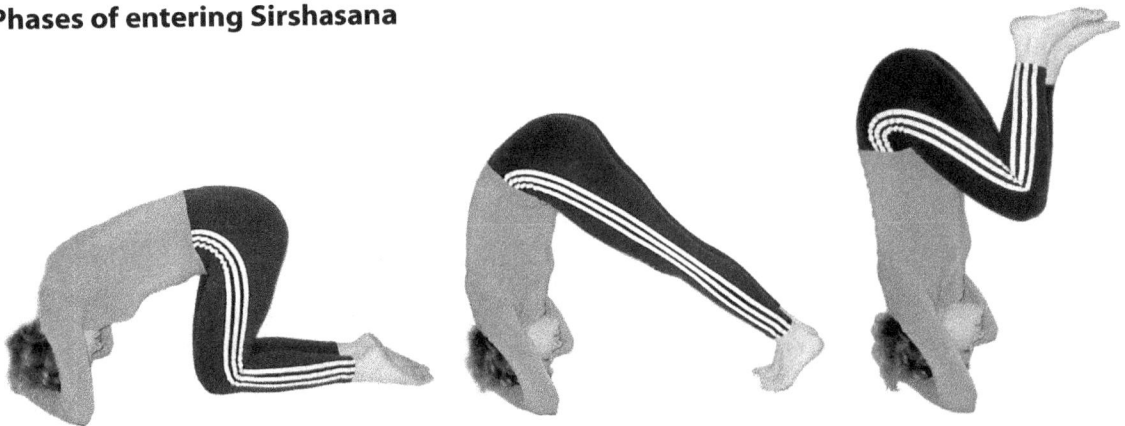

126

Sirshasana's variations

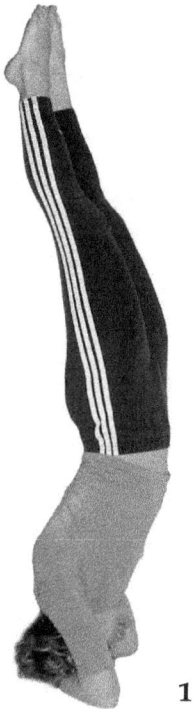

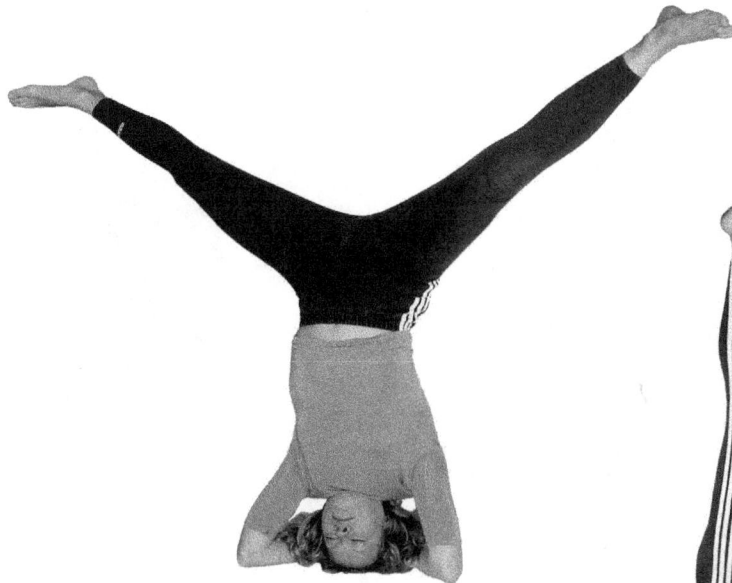

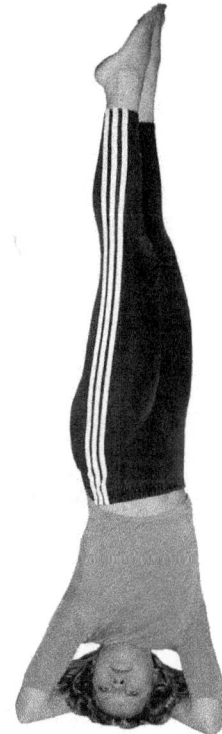

Variations of Sirshasana:

1 — Kapalasana (Sirshasana with arching); 2 — Sirshasana with legs apart; 3 — Sirshasana with pivoted spine

Squeezing out asanas

Maiurasana
(peacock pose)

Maiurasana is a squeezing out pose that should be done with the straight back. The energy you squeeze out from the lower part (Manipura and pancreas) moves like in Bhujangasana. It can be replaced: like a stretching pose — by bhujangasana; and like a squeezing pose — by lying face down on the wrists under the belly (which is a good help, if you overate). If you can't do asana well, better don't do it at all.

Gomukhasana
(bull's head pose)

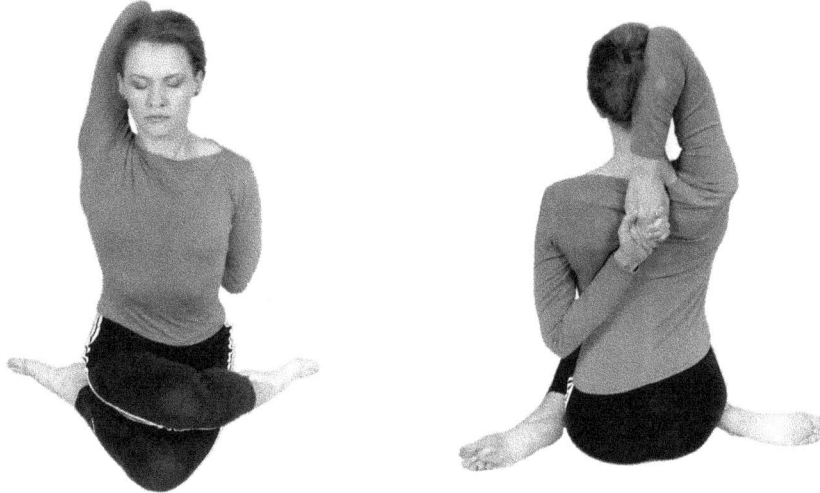

Advanced strengthening poses

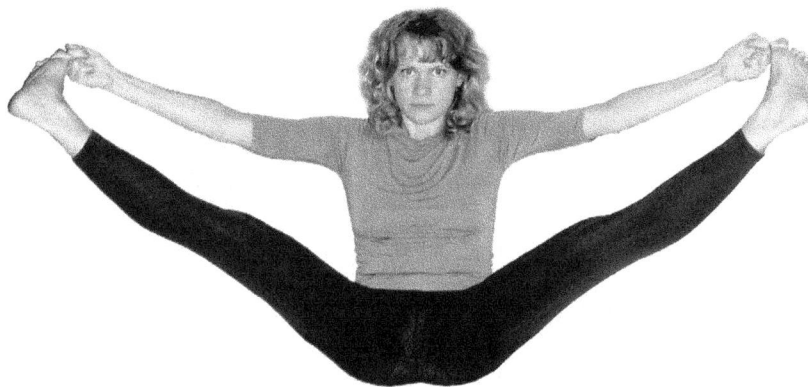

**Merundandasana
(mountain Meru or the vertebral column pose)**

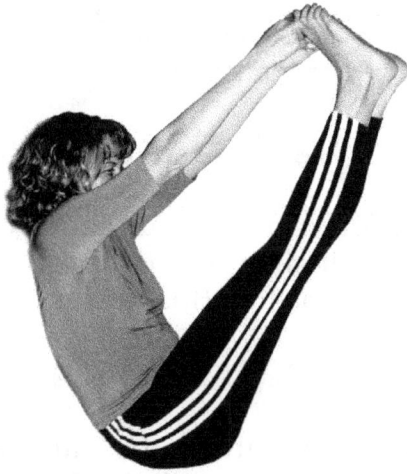

**Niralamba-Pashimottanasana
(stretching back without
support pose)**

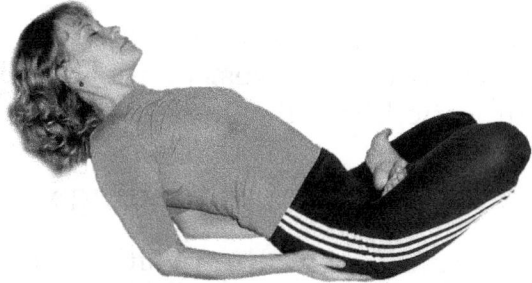

Tolangulasana (scale pose)

Equilibration poses

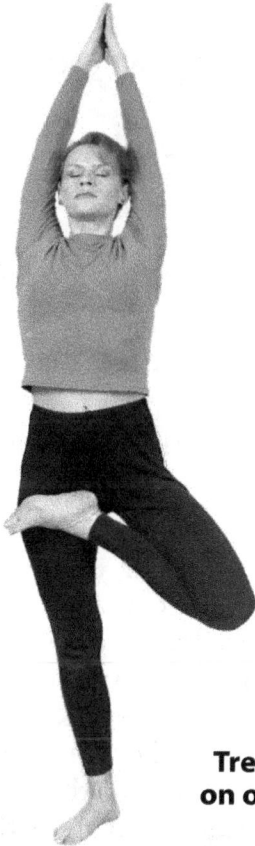

**Padangushthasana
(tiptoe pose)**

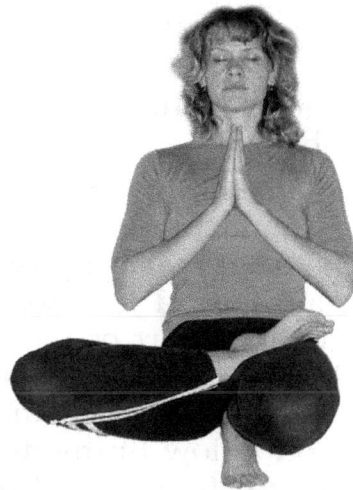

**Tree pose
on one foot**

Advanced pranayamas

Bhastrika and its variations

The physiological effect from Bhastrika can vary depending on the position of the eyes, of the head, or by closing one of the nostrils (asymmetric Bhastrikas). Hence there are six types of Bhastrikas.

«Standing» Bhastrikas

They differ by the position of the body, in which they are done. The technique is the same, which is the common Bhastrika.

1. In standing position, hands in namaste, the head is straight, eyes are open and focused on the point on the floor, situated in about 1,5 m from your toes, i.e. looking at the angle of 45° down.

   ATTENTION! In this technique it's crucial to squint eyes without moving your head.

2. In standing position, hands in namaste, the head dropped back. Eyes are open and focused between eyebrows.

   ATTENTION! a) the head should be dropped back only by the neck, not the back; b) posterior muscles of the neck must be relaxed.

3. In standing position, hands in namaste, the head and the neck in relaxed djalanadhara bandha. Eyes are open and focused on the wings of nose.

   ATTENTION! The back of the neck must be stretched and the anterior part as relaxed as possible.

4. Position like in 2, but open eyes are focused on the wings of nose.

Remember, that after the intensive breathing of Bhastrika, it's crucial to do kumbhaka.

Effects and action. Like a basic Bhastrika, these variations provide hyperventilation and the inside hydraulic massage. However different positions of the head make it possible to control blood inflow and outflow to the head. Indeed the blood flows into the head by arteries, located on the anterior part of the neck, whereas the natural (valveless) drainage — through the venous system in the back of the neck. The stretching of the relative zone makes the blood flow weaker and enhanced the blood inflow (in the third variation) or its outflow (the 2nd and the 4th). This is training not only the vascular system, but also the adapting capacities of the brain.

«Asymmetric» Bhastrikas

The action of asymmetric Bhastrikas relies on making airflow denser by reducing the admission section of the airway, like in Akapalabhati.

First variation

Starting position. Like in Akapalabhati, i.e. the giving hand in yoni mudra near the nose.

Technique. The breathing is done like in Bhastrika, but through one nostril.

After finishing half of the cycle, change the nostril.

Second variation

The same as in previous, but inhale through one nostril and exhale through another.

Bramari (the bee)

Bramari is a vibration pranayama.

Starting position. Any meditative posture.

Technique. Inhaling, hum with your nose, like a bee by tonality. Exhaling (still by the nose), hum in one tone lower. In both cases there must be a physical vibration in the skull (in different zones of the head).

Anuloma viloma

This exercise is one of the most important in coming from hatha yoga to it's more advanced levels. Nevertheless it should be mastered gradually.

First step

Sit in a meditative asana. The giving hand in yoni mudra, the taking one — in dhiana mudra. Breathing rhythmically, close one nostril after another by this scheme: inhale by the left nostril, exhale by the right one, inhale by the right nostril, exhale by the left one. Men should start by the left nostril, women — by the right one. Breathing rhythm should be natural. The exercise should be done for at least 10 minutes.

Second step

Adding breath holds (see «Exercises with breath holds»).

Third step

Adding energy work (see chapter «Techniques of work with energy»).

Advanced elements of warming-up

At the advanced level or with the better physical development the warming-up can be enhanced to become more efficient. First of all I recommend to start with a self-massage (usual and a pointillage), and after warming-up the joints to add some aerobic exercises, working out the cardio-vascular system, and in addition to that some exercises to warm-up viscera (bandhas and kriyas), voice warm-up (simhasana) and dynamic complexes Suria Namaskar (in a sunny time of the day) and Chandra Namaskar (especially good at a full moon).

Self-massage

The self-massage can include a contact and non-contact facials, massage of ears, head, neck, viscera of abdominal cavity, of legs and arms.

Warm-up enhancers

Those practitioners, who are used to all warming-up exercises, can look at their fingers. There is a simple test: stretch your arms before you, your fingers straight, and hold for some time. Gradually you'll see that some of your fingers automatically folder. Those fingers that crook less are the less energised. So the respective meridians are weakened as well. In this case, warming-up palms, you should pay special attention to these fingers and musculotendinous meridians. An additional effect can be achieved, if you clench the wrists or make a mudra during the warm-up. **The warm-up should be done with Muladhara set-up,** i.e. with the feeling, working out tendons.

The simplest way to enhance the legs warming-up is to raise legs higher than usual. The tension rises according to the angle. Another alternative is to draw the leg aside, turning it — in this way other muscles are worked-out. Depending on the angle of drawing the leg, we can activate different musculotendinous meridians.

Bandhas and kriyas

Bandhas and kriyas are done either as separate exercises or together with asanas and pranayamas. They can also be used as warm-up elements. Because they work with viscera, it's logical to do them in the end of warming-up («from periphery to the centre»).

132

Mulabandha

Starting position. This exercise can be done practically in any position. In warming-up it's ok to do it standing, but the biggest effect it gives in padmasana (lotus posture, not even the half-lotus), because groin muscles are specially stretched. The rest of starting positions make no difference.

Technique. Concurrently squeeze your muscles of the anus sphincter, the pelvic floor and of the genitals. This exercise can be done in the quick tempo or with long holding of muscles.

Inside criteria of doing mulabandha correctly is the feeling that all viscera «rise».

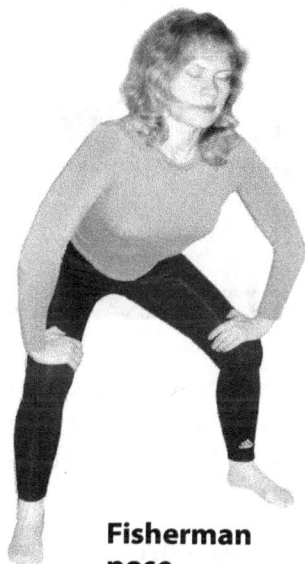

Fisherman pose

Uddiana bandha (fisherman pose)

Starting position. This pose makes exercises easier, taking off the tension from the belly.

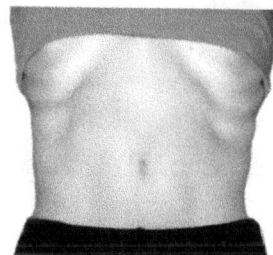

Technique. Exhale fully, drawing your belly «to the spine», slightly lifting it to the ribs. Sometimes it makes sense to do djvaladhara and Muladhara bandhas at the same time. Inhaling, exit the fisherman's pose, relaxing your belly. Uddiana bandha is usually repeated three times in a row.

Particularities. As it was already said, the inhalation should last as long as the exhalation. There is no need to do bandha till everything goes dark before your eyes and then to gasp for some air. The time of doing should let you do the inhalation with no rush.

The action of bandhas is described above.

Uddiana bandha kriya

Starting position. As in the previous exercise.

Technique. After taking uddiana bandha relax your abdominal muscles, so that your belly «falls out». Repeat several times, accelerating tempo. Ideally raise it with the speed up to 2 times a second. However it's more important to find your our rhythm and to change tempo so that you don't get habituation.

Nauli

Starting position. Fisherman's pose.

Technique. Draw your belly in and throw out the rectus, then try to revolve it. Once this muscle comes out, there will be no more problems. Your back must be straight — it helps the energy to go up.

Criteria. While doing nauli one must feel the heat lifting.

Particularities. In the first phase of doing this exercise you should hold the djanaladhara bandha, otherwise the energy can move from the head down. When the heat reaches the throat, djalanhara bandha should be unlocked to let the energy come to the head. In this case there is a feeling of «enlightenment» in the eyes, i.e. as if everything became clearer. This feeling determines the duration of this exercise for everyone personally.

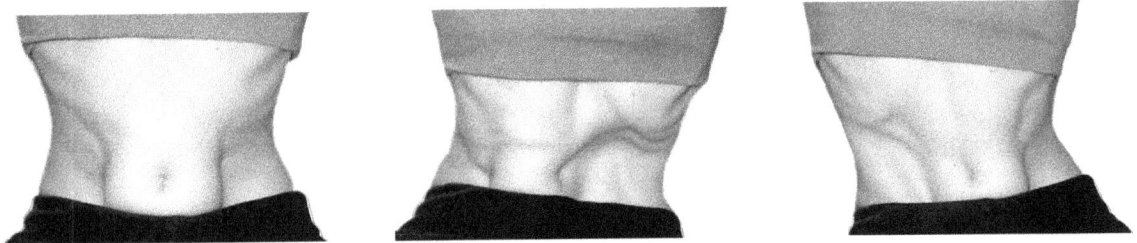

WARNING!. Nauli raises the male[1] sexual energy. In this case it is useful for those who practice brahmacharia or sex without ejaculation — it preserves from congestion causing prostatitis, but, if you don't drive the energy to the head, it easily falls back almost out of control.

Uddiana bandha, uddiana bandha kriya and nauli can be considered as hygienic gymnastics, good for everyday practice. **Exercises done in series, men should do odd times and women even times.**

Respiratory warm-up

Simhasana (lion pose)

This exercise is good to do in warming-up after nauli, because at this moment the energy is raised up.

Starting position. Standing or sitting.

Technique. Do a full yoga inhalation. Firmly press the tip of your tongue to the upper palate, so that the throat would be strained. Drawing your head and your neck ahead, do some full rotation movements

---

[1]   For women the same effect is done by viparita karani.

134

by your head. If you're doing it correctly, the tension in muscles moves in the neck ring — when head is up, the tension is down and vice versa. Stick out your tongue as far as you can, so that you feel tension in the throat and in the back of your tongue) and let out a roar like that of a lion. Roar till the air leaves your lungs. Holding the breath after the exhalation, again press your tongue to the palate and rotate your head.

Action. It is easy to see by one's own experience, that pressing the tongue to the palate, we strain our muscles of the throat that usually almost never get strained. Rotating the head, we «drive» this tension around: when the head is up, the lower, anterior zone of the throat gets strained, and vice versa. The higher the tongue is pressed (to the teeth, to the near palate, to the far palate), the deeper zones are activated. So the first and the last stages of the exercise provide the inside massage of the throat by the muscle tension — there is no other way to massage this zone, because it is out of access.

The roar should be done not by the throat, not by vocal ligaments, but with the whole inside, as if doing the vibration massage. Roaring with the throat, you'll just strain your voice and get no effect. To do the exercise right, you must not just show your tongue, but stretch it out at the maximum. Note that **the farther you stretch out your tongue (being relaxed), the deeper your larynx gets strained.** This makes it possible to vary the therapeutic effect from this asana.

There is a variation of simhasana, where the tongue is stretched not down, but up. It helps to activate some throat muscles that are not used in our everyday life. In this asana the neck should be strained in the posterior part, then the effect will come.

Maha mudra (the great mudra)

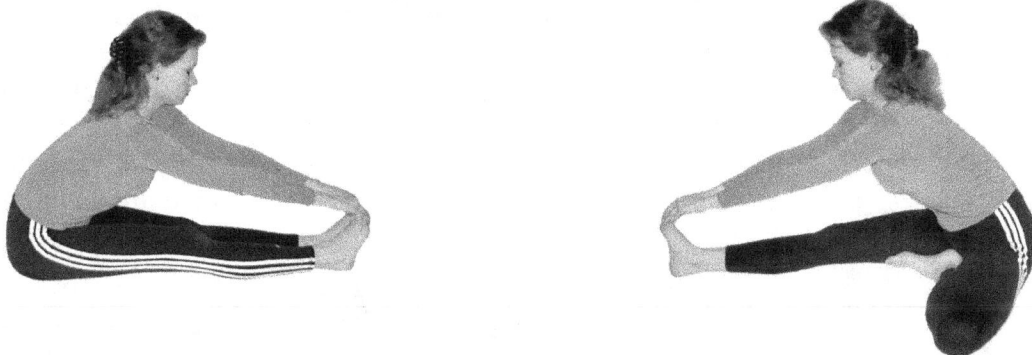

ATTENTION! Unlike Pashimottanasana, maha mudra is done with the straight back. The bending is done only by the pelvis. Mudra is done with three bandhas and holding the breath after inhalation. This is an advanced exercise. **I don't recommend practicing it without additional clues from your Teacher.**

Suria Namaskar
(«Salutation to the Sun» complex)

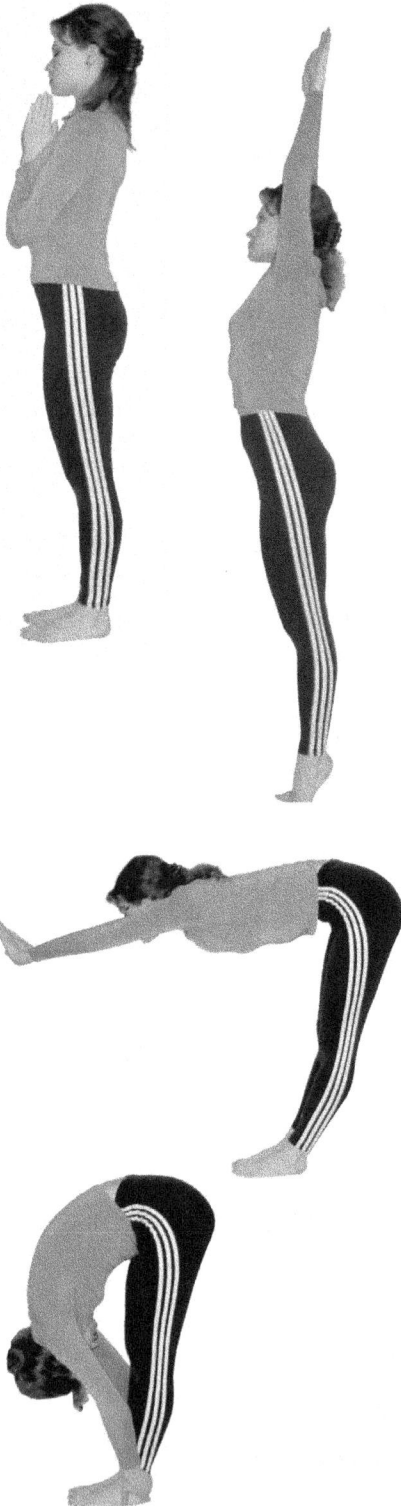

1. Pranamasana (praying pose)

Stand still and straight. Face the Sun or its direction (if it is hidden by the clouds). Put your hands together in the namaste position. Close your eyes and relax. Actualise your body for at least half a minute. This will prepare you for the practice. Try consciously to relax all the muscles of your body. Breath: some full yoga breathings.

2. Hasta Uttanasana (raised hands pose)

Inhaling, raise your hands above the head, at the same time standing on tiptoes. In the final position hands are straight in the elbows and parallel to each other; palms ahead. Continue rhythmic breathing.

3. Padahastasana (stork pose)

Exhaling, carefully come down on your full feet, bend ahead and put your hands on the floor before your feet or grab your ankles. All the movement should be fluent with no jerks. The bending should start at lower vertebra and go to the top — as in Pashimottanasana. Try to keep your legs straight. If possible, try to touch your knees with the forehead or the chin. Continue rhythmic breathing.

People with the stiff back (lower back) may find it difficult to achieve the perfect form of padahastasana. They should work on the constant strain in the posterior part of the body: from toes till the crown of the head.

136

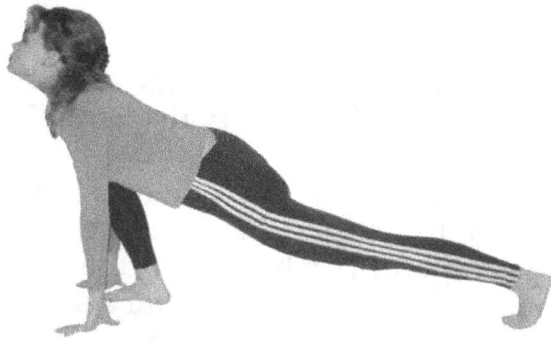

4. Ashva Sanchalasana (horseman pose)

Inhaling, draw back your right (left for women) leg — sliding on the floor, as far as possible. At the same time bend you left knee, keeping the left foot at the same place (in other words, do the left knee lunge ahead), arching from the upper vertebra to the lower ones (as in Bhujangasana). Hands touch the floor, elbows are straight.

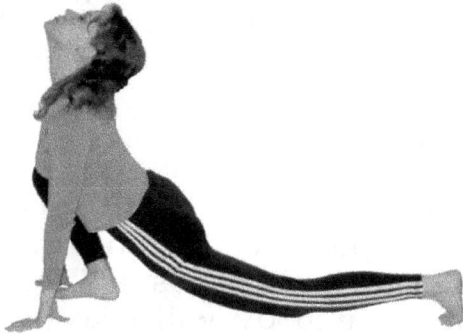

5. Parvatasana (mountain pose)

Exhaling, take the right knee off the floor, at the same time dropping the head forward. Straightening the body in the lower back, stretch the left leg back (straightening the knee at the same time with taking the right leg off the floor) and put both feet together. You will end up in the «set» position, which is the mountain pose.

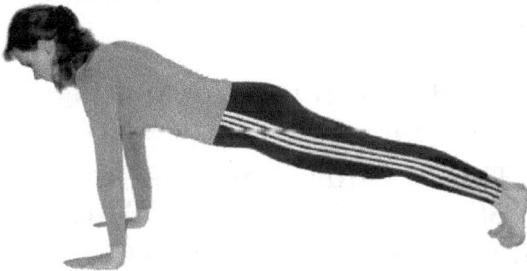

6. Ashtanga Namaskar (worship on eight points)

This posture is called like this because in the final position the body touches the floor in eight points. This pose is also called «zigzag».

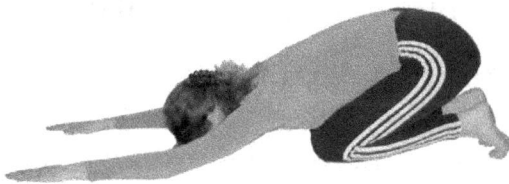

Exhaling go down on all fours, slightly touch the floor by the forehead, moving forward your head and the body. In the end of this movement, let the chest slide on the floor and put your chin on the ground. In the final position eight points must touch the floor: chin, chest, both hands, both knees and the toes.

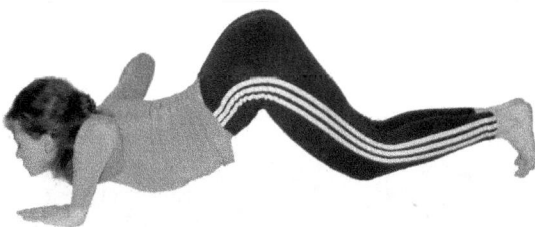

137

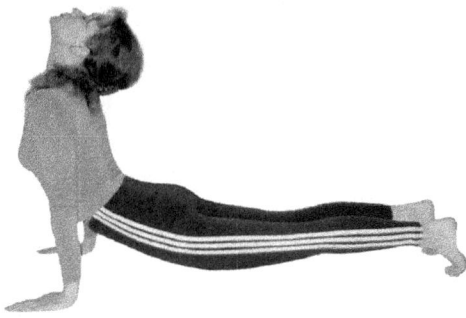

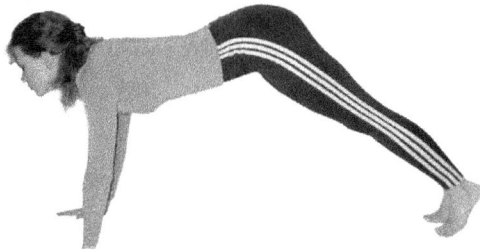

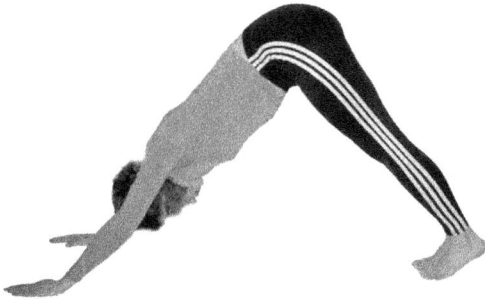

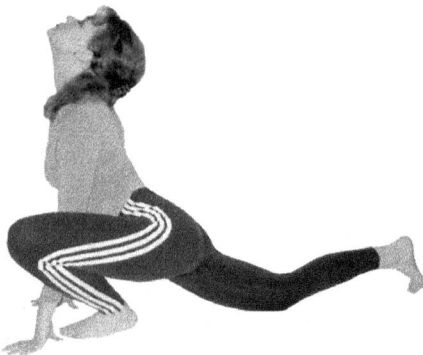

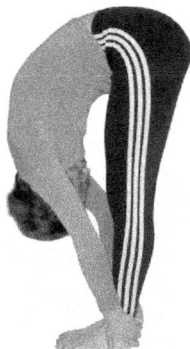

7. Dog pose

Inhaling, continue the zigzag-like movement of the body, straightening your arms so that the lower back arches. The movement should go from the top down. In the final position the upper body and the head must be dropped back as far as possible and comfortable. Knees don't touch the ground. Coming into this pose from the previous one, hands and feet must stay in the same position.

8. Cat pose

Exhaling, lift your pelvis as high as possible, keeping the same position of your hands and feet. As a result, your body will take the arch-like position. The arms and the back must form one straight line. The legs are straight.

9. Ashva Sanchalasana (horseman pose)

This posture mirrors number four of Suria Namaskar. Bend the left knee, put the foot between your hands. At the same time lift your head up (as in the exercise 4, but in the mirror way) and so on. The pose is also entered with the **inhalation**.

10. Padahastasana

Is a repeating of the 3nd exercise. Also done with an **exhalation**.

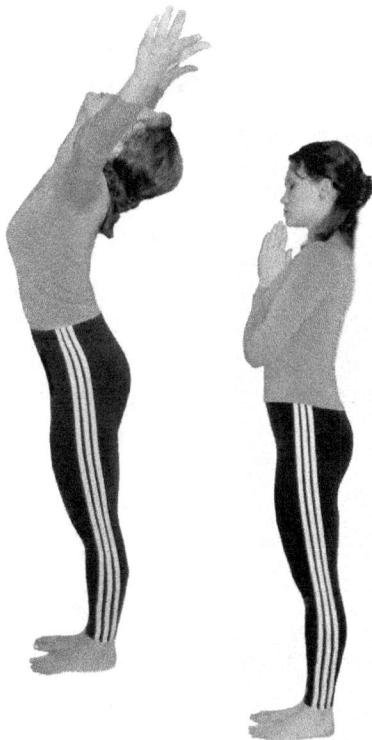

11. Hasta Uttanasana

This pose is similar to the 2nd posture of SN, only there is no need to stand on tiptoes, instead you should arch the back in the zone of your heart.

The pose is done with an **inhalation**.

12. Pranamasana (praying pose)

It's the final position, similar to the first one. Taking this pose you should **exhale**. Staying in this position breathe rhythmically till you continue your practice (start doing next cycle of Suria Namaskar).

Comments on practicing Suria Namaskar

All exercises are done in one breathing rhythm. Movements should be done according to breathing and not vice versa. Every movement must be smooth and fully conscious. In every pose several cycles of rhythmic breathing should be done.

Some small pranayamas

Small pranayamas aren't very typical for yoga and aren't used by all Schools. Legend has it that small pranayamas were found by one of the Teachers in an old library. However small because pranayamas aren't mentioned in the original yoga sources I know, I suppose they were taken from another system. Because of their Manipura martial character, most probably they come from martial arts schools, which were in abundance presented in India. Doing small pranayamas you should pay attention to the following three clues.

1. Pranayamas should be done with Manipura set-up.

2. Exercises are done at a breath hold. All the particularities of performing kumbhaka (as indicated above) should be taken into account.

3. Arms in pranayamas 1, 2, 3, 7, 8 should be straight in elbows, shoulders down. This pose drives energy to Anahata. Otherwise exercises lose the most of its effect (see warming-up in the chapter «First steps in hatha-yoga»).

Pranayama № 1 (tree)

Starting position. Standing, feet together, hands down long the body.

Technique. With the full yoga inhalation raise your arms by sides to joint your hands above the head. Elbows should be straight, all the body stretched from the tips of fingers to toes. Do kumbhaka. Exhaling, put your hands down in the reverse order. Inhalation should be as long as exhalation.

Pranayama № 2 (skier)

Starting position. Standing, feet together, hands down long the body.

Technique. With a full yoga inhalation, raise your straight arms before yourself, hands clenched in wrists. With kumbhaka do some energetic flap motions by your arms going up and down to the highest degree. They should move synchronously, parallel to each other. Avoid folding your elbows (typical for breached Anahata). As soon as the breath-hold becomes uncomfortable, return your arms in the position parallel to the floor and do the «kha» exhalation. Put your arms down.

Pranayama № 3 (mill)

Starting position. Standing, feet together, hands down long the body.

Technique. With the full yoga inhalation raise the straight arms before yourself, the middle and the index fingers pressed by the thumb, little finger and the ring finger straight. Do kumbhaka. One arm goes backwards (to make the angle between hands 180°). Synchronously rotate your arms by the shoulder joint (keeping clavicles still). End up as in previous exercise.

This pranayama relaxes the shoulder girdle.

Pranayama № 4

In this pranayama you should push up from the floor, holding kumbhaka. Take off the breath-hold, exhaling «kha».

Pranayama № 7 (hammer)

Starting position. Standing, feet apart, wider than shoulders.

Technique. With the full yoga inhalation raise your straight arms by the sides to join them above the head in a lock. Holding kumbhaka, rotate your body, rocking more and more the lower back (as always vertebra after vertebra). Having reached the widest amplitude of turning the whole body, gradually diminish the amplitude, stopping rotation from the bottom up. When the rotation is over, exhale with «kha».

Pranayama № 8

Starting position. Standing, feet apart, wider than shoulders.

Technique. With the full yoga inhalation raise the straight arms before yourself. Clench the fists and do kumbhaka. Sharply move your hands apart, «opening» your chest to the full. Join your hands by the wrists before yourself (central position). Leaving one hand before yourself, turn your body back and put another hand behind yourself, the head turned to the back hand (i.e. look back). Come back to the central position. Do the same thing for the other side. Continue the cycle until kumbhaka is over. Exhale with a «kha».

> **NOTE.** Turn your body just by pivoting your spine. Keep your elbows straight. Motion is energetic with Manipura set-up.

Pranayama № 10 (breathing for steady nerves)

Starting position. Standing, feet together or slightly apart.

Technique. Inhale with FYB, raising the arms before yourself till the level of shoulders, palms up. Clench fists, hold your breath and with an effort (as if overcoming the inside resistance) fold your arms in elbows. The same way, with an effort, unfold them. As soon as your arms unfold parallel to the floor, immediately relax them and, relaxed, fold them quickly again. Unfold with an effort. Repeat this cycle several times. Finish exhaling «kha».

In this exercise nerves are steadied by quick changing of tension/ relaxation. Indeed, **the healthier your nerve system is, the wider your scope of states: from the extreme tension to the extreme relaxation and the rest.** The problem person finds it difficult both to relax completely and to strain strongly. Making this scope wider is one of yoga's goals.

Pranayama № 11 (waking up lung cells)

Starting position. Standing.

Technique. Inhale with FYB and start striking your chest with tense fingers from bottom up. Holding breath, massage the thorax. Exhaling, repeat the striking. This pranayama intensifies the blood flow in lung alveolus, improving respiratory metabolism and make the phlegm cough out. That's is why after this pranayama you should cough. It also relaxes thorax muscles.

Variation. Striking is done more intensively — with fists. Exhaling, hum with the open mouth. This variation of pranayama helps «to open» vocal resonators.

Gymnastics to «cleanse» musculotendinous meridians (MTM)

The principle of cleansing MTM is the same we used in asanas: to open a channel we must consequently stretch it to pass the strain long all the channel.

1. Cleansing pericardium

Starting position. Standing, hands long the body. Palms and fingers are straight and parallel to the floor. Inhaling, hold this position of fingers and raise your arms by sides, so that the tension goes by the inner side of arms from the fingers down to the ribs.

Criteria. This exercise is effective, only if fingers are strained at the maximum, elbows are straight and shoulders aren't lifted. All these conditions are difficult to do (as well as very useful) for people with depressed Anahata and the problem meridian. Where the tension disappears, the channel is «clogged».

2. Cleansing of three heaters meridian

Starting position. The same, but the hands are clenched in fists, twisted in order that the back of the palm is parallel to the floor.

Technique is the same as in previous exercise.

3. Cleansing of the heart

Starting position. Standing, hands apart parallel to the floor, fingers stretched out.

Technique. Inhaling, twist your palms, so that the tension would go from the little finger up the hand to the chest.

4. Cleansing of lungs meridian

The same as in the previous, but the strain should go from the thumb to the intraclavicular hollow.

5. Cleansing of rectum

As in the exercise 3, but clenching fists. The tension goes from the index knuckle to the neck.

6. Cleansing of small intestine.

I propose to my reader to find techniques of cleansing six leg meridians on his own, taking as a base the described principle and MTM schemes, given in Appendix 1.

142

PRINCIPLES OF BUILDING YOGA COMPLEXES

Let's take a look on principles of building yoga complexes, which would help advanced readers make their own complexes. Note that **these principles are meant for relatively healthy people, who practice yoga to increase their energy and for their spiritual growth.** The principles of building therapeutic complexes will be overlooked in one of the next coming chapters.

Principle of compensation

By the example of the given basic complexes we learned about the primary principle of building these complexes — the principle of compensation. It means that every next asana compensates the effect from the previous one. For example, Bhujangasana activates ANS and lifts the energy to the head, and pashimmatanasana that follows it, smoothes the energy and drives it downwards. After this complex we return to our primary state, only at a higher energy level. Minor anomalies of the state are compensated, because in the «swirling» energy different «holes» in the etheric body and smoothes «bumps» itself. Our body chooses itself the needed influence, like it chooses the needed active elements from the medical mixture, containing components with opposite action.

Building complex at a principle of compensation is the safest way for beginners, because all undesirable or excessive influences of asanas (like the additional raising of blood pressure for a hypertensive patient) are compensated by asanas with the opposite action. When the practitioner develops a good sense of his body, he can vary the duration of each asana according to his needs.

Principle of enhancing (swirling the energy)

As it was already said, there are six categories of asanas: stretching, pivoting, strengthening, squeezing, inverted and equilibration. Besides asanas can be divided into four groups according to the direction of the spine to the line of the horizon.

Each channel can be worked out in four planes, which explains **the principle of similitude of asanas.** For example, Bhujangasana works with the anterior-middle channel in the horizontal plane, Ushtrasana — the same channel in the vertical plane (turning for 90°), Chakrasana — the belly up (90° more) and the scorpion pose work out the same meridian with the turn of 270°. Another example: Pashimmatanasana, Padahastasana, Halasana and Pindasana within Sirshasana (asana standing on the head, feet close to the head) work out the posterior-middle channel in four planes. The quartet of pivoting asanas is: Arthamatsiendrasana, Trikonasana, parsva Sirshasana (standing on the head with the pivoted spine), Parivritta Parsvakonasana.

It's easy to notice that asanas become more intensive with every plane, which together with the principle of compensation defines the method of joining them into a complex.

Every next group of asanas must include asanas working with the same plane and should be balanced as for its action. Groups of asanas must aim at the consequent work with all four planes up till the highest possible (as for the level of difficulty of exercises).

The nature of enhancing of the effect from each next group has to do with the gravity. For example, the stretching in padahastasana is stronger than in pashimmatanasana, because the body reaches for the earth more, thanks to the gravity. Like in Ushtrasana the strain is enhanced by the gravity, while in Bhujangasana it should be overcome to create a strain.

Besides, changing the plane, we can activate the humoral effect from exercises.

Principle of «swinging»

The principles of building yoga complexes, described above, are based on the consequent compensation of each asana's action, causing the relatively insignificant «swinging» of the activity of our ANS — from asana to asana. Such an approach is quite safe, which allows using it in the practice for beginners. However more advanced practitioners

144

with the good health, who «got used» to compensated complexes, can find more useful a more complicated approach to build yoga complex. The «swinging» principle implies doing more and more difficult exercises of the same group (for example, Bhujangasana — Ushtrasana — dhanurasana and so on), which is afterwards compensated by a group of contrary asanas (Pashimottanasana — Padahastasana — Halasana and so on). Then the scope of «swinging» of ANS (as well as the grade of its training) is much bigger than in previous methods.

Principle of using the elements in yoga complexes

Different types of exercises correspond with different elements, activated in our body. Let's analyse this connection at the example of yoga complexes given above (see chapter «First steps in hatha yoga»).

In each complex there are blocks, which have to do with basic elements, at least with five of them. For instance, the warming-up brings the element of the Wood, it wakes our body from the yin, passive, sleepy state, making our blood flow faster etc.

Small pranayamas correspond to fire element, they are done with Manipura set-up, tone us, raise our blood pressure and intensify the blood flow. Asanas in our interpretation (there can be others), correspond to the element of Water.

Big pranayamas correspond to Air element, which with some admission equals the Metal in Chinese tradition. Indeed, Akapalabhati, Kapalabhati, anuloma viloma, Bhastrika — all pranayamas done by lungs, pump air into our body on the other hand cool our lungs (putting us from yang state into yin).

Strengthening asanas firm us and correspond to Earth element.

Coordination of practice with weather

When we do a yoga complex, we must activate all elements, except for the case when one of them is excessive in nature.

For example, if you practice, when it's hot, there is no need to stress yourself with small pranayamas, because there is already a lot of Fire around, so there's no need to get it more. The excess of Fire starts destroying Water and Wood in our body — we start sweating and can eventually have a heat stroke.

Fire

Wood

Earth

Water

Metal

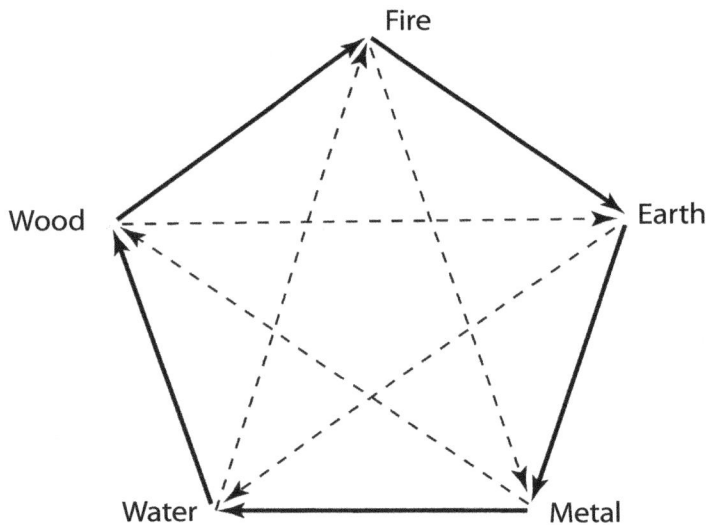

Or, if you are doing yoga in a wet cold day, asanas should be limited, because, if you add Water to your body, your state will aggravate — there will be heaviness in the body. The warming-up, joints gymnastics is on the contrary good for a wet weather, because Wood makes yang out of yin.

In a cold wet weather it's not recommended to do many small pranayamas either, because excessive Fire will confront water, overstressing your cardio-vascular system.

For the same reason it's not good to practice big pranayamas in high humidity, i.e. at the excessive Water, because Air (or else Metal) produces Water (pure Yin), cooling the body. Physically this cooling is done when air comes into our lungs.

Taking into account the balance of elements in your environment and in yourself, you can build yoga complexes to bring all elements into a perfect harmony.

Their disbalance can cause unpleasant aspects. For example, if you do just asanas with no warm-up, you get the feeling of «clogged» joints, you body will feel heavy, because Water, the basic element of Yin, is heavy and to compensate it you must activate Yang aspects.

If you practice big pranayamas in the windy weather, you'll get too much Air element together with the dizziness, looseness, you'll be reeling, because this element isn't compensated.

In the open air the balance of elements is different than indoors, so «home yogins» sometimes find it difficult to practice outdoors. So the complex must be built differently. In the open air the density of

146

natural etheric energies is higher and the effect of saturation comes faster than indoors. Besides there are outer flows of energy, which can hamper the conscious work with energy. For example, if you sit your side to the sun, you'll find it difficult to take the energy from the front side, because all the flows you create will be «swept off» by the sun energy.

Speaking about the influence of the environment and weather on your optimal complex, don't forget about the importance of the barometric pressure. When it is low, it makes sense to compensate the languor by starting you session with the accent on activating anterior stretching asanas — such as Bhujangasana; while at a high pressure it's OK to start with yoga mudra and to make an accent on the stretching back and relaxing asanas.

Principle of following the body (free complex)

This principle is the highest, the most efficient and, actually, the most advanced level of yoga practice. It means that actualising the needs of your physical body (and as a result, of your etheric body), the practitioner **does asanas, which his body demands,** by natural mechanisms of body's self-control. It may seem that this method is so natural that one may not need no others and start studying yoga immediately from this, but unfortunately it's not that easy.

Tell a group of people to do some natural movements, imposed by their body (as in Osho's *latihana*[1]) and look at them. You'll immediately see that their movements don't come «freely» and naturally. On the contrary, everyone is doing the cycle of stereotype movements, leading in most cases to no catharsis. Their movements only seem free, but in fact undercover from the consciousness, they are controlled... by the consciousness! And not by the body.

The same can happens in yoga. An inexperienced practitioner can find the following obstacles to practice yoga naturally:

1. Incapacity to actualise the natural needs of the body. Most of adults find it very difficult to actualise their real needs, changing the actualisation by a habit. If it weren't so, harmful self-destructing habits as smoking, drinking and unhealthy diet would disappear themselves.

---

[1] To be more precise, latihan is a Sufi technique, but in the dance interpretation, as it became known to modern practitioners, it was given by Osho.

2. Half-conscious, following the unwillingness to work (in the spiritual meaning) striving to do only those poses, he can do well, but according to the principle of similarity of physical and energetic postures, these asanas are the less needed for the body.

3. Demonstration — i.e. the wish (also unconscious) to look good in doing yoga postures, to the prejudice of the real needs of the body.

4. Suggestibility — unconscious wish to do what the colleague in the gym or the instructor does.

5. Personal dynamic stereotypes, which can happen, if people used to practice in a «canonical» school. Starting a free complex, they quickly finish by doing one of their usual complexes.

In other words, the free following of the body should be practice after you are sure to actualise your real and not foreign wishes.

Practicing in groups you should remember that this practice doesn't form a common flow, that's why the practitioner may find its effect weaker.

I recommend starting the natural yoga session in the middle of the second year in addition to standard complexes, «warming-up» by the common flow, and after the third year make it the main method.

Sequence of doing pranayamas

For beginners the most efficient sequence of pranayamas is the one when chakras are worked out from the top down. It has to do with the fact that the air passes the respiratory tract from the top down. The optimal sequence for beginners is: Kapalabhati, ujai, bramari, kumbhaka, Bhastrika, anuloma viloma, sukh-purak.

As it was said above, pranayamas secure the effect from asanas, energizing the formed posture. On the other hand pranayamas are more efficient, if done after cleansing the channels by asanas. Understanding these principles forms the idea that we can build a complex, where asanas and pranayamas would take turns. For example, experienced practitioners can be advised the following method of work with problem zones and situations. Do a couple of asanas, working out the chakra from the front, a couple of asanas working out the chakra from the back, one asana to work the diagonal meridian, like described in the chapter «First steps in hatha yoga». After that, do respiratory exercises, securing the corresponding effect at the needed chakra. Then pass to another chakra.

Cumulative routines

Some exercises make the effect from each other much stronger, if done in sequences. The effect can be even greater, if the sequence is done several times. Here are some examples of cumulative routines: «activation of lung cells» — Simhasana; yoga-mudra — Kapalabhati.

Accordance of asanas and pranayamas

As mentioned above, pranayamas strengthen asanas effect, energizing the upbuilding that was made by them. On the other hand, pranayama effect is more evident if they are performed after cleanhing channels with asanas. Understanding of these principles brings forward the idea of the possibility of building up complexes, where asanas and pranayamas are «mixed» with each other. For example, for experienced practitioners it is possible to recommend the following scheme of working with problematic areas and problematic situations. One or two asanas are performed to work out the chakra from the front side; one or two that work the chakra out from the back side; one, working it out as described in chapter «First steps in Hatha-yoga». Next, breathing exercises are done to stabilize respective effect in respective chakra. Then one can move on to the next chakra.

Accents in breathing

If doing a yoga complex you feel a need to nurture one of the chakras, you can practice breathing on this chakra. Note that depending on if we want to stimulate a chakra (pump it in) or «cleanse» it (take off the excessive energy), we should focus on inhaling or on exhaling. Especially good results are done by accenting on inhaling or on exhaling while doing such exercises as Kapalabhati and Bhastrika. Meditative images that can be used to form breathing of different types, have to do with the feeling of a «non-stop» filling of lungs or on the contrary, emptying them. Just «occasionally» they are interrupted by the contrary phase of breathing.

Accenting of the breathing on a chakra can be enhanced by the practice of the articulated pronunciation of chakra-mantras. You can see that this exercise is done right, if in FYB the needed chakra is heating.

ASANAS WITH BREATH-HOLDS (ADVANCED LEVEL)

How breath-holds influence the body

Asanas accompanied with holding breath is the advanced level technique, because breath-holds imply a good physical health and the adequate self-analysis of your state. If a person practices breath-holds having no strong cardio-vascular system, no healthy lungs etc. he can once and for all «injure» his heart.

Breath-holds enhance the general effect of asana on the body, first of all on the cardio-vascular system. Besides, **holding breath after inhaling intensifies the energy moving up and raises the blood pressure; while holding breath after exhaling intensifies the energy going down and lowers the BP.** Using this principle with the help of breath-holds we can make energy move more intensively up or down, of course, if asana is done correctly.

There are three types of breathing with holds: «inhaling», «exhaling» and mixed.

«Inhaling» breath is done like this: **inhale-hold-exhale.** The rhythm of inhaling, holding and exhaling should make it possible to keep this breathing as long as you want, once you started it right — like the rhythmic breathing. You should find a natural rhythm, corresponding your physiological cycle, and then try to build it at this scheme. Then you will be sure that you»ve chosen the right breathing, if you can keep this rhythm for a long time, and after 5-6 breathings you don't need to catch your breath. To begin you should inhale and exhale as in FYB, making a short hold in between, just for some seconds.

«Exhaling» breathing formula is **exhale-hold-inhale.** «Exhaling» breath calms down, lowers the blood pressure and makes energy move down.

150

Coordination of asanas with breath-holds

Basing on principles how energy moves, we can understand how to use these types of breathing in complexes. The effect of asanas, which are entered with inhaling (i.e. anterior arching poses, making energy go up, like *Bhujangasana, Ushtrasana, Dhanurasana etc.*) is enhanced by a «inhaling» breath in the asana.

On the contrary such asanas as *yoga mudra, Pashimottanasana, Padahastasana, Halasana* are done with the «exhale» breathing, because they naturally drive the energy downwards, so breathing like this, we make this effect stronger.

So with the help of breath-holds we intensify energy's movement up or down.

> **ATTENTION!** These techniques strongly influence the blood pressure, so, if you have problems with it, you should be careful. If you already have a high pressure, «inhaling» breath shouldn't be done, likewise with the low pressure you can't practice the «exhaling» breath. The contrary is also true — both breathings can be perfectly used as therapeutic techniques.

Breathing with holds, like all other respiratory exercises, should be done in the individual rhythm, i.e. the ratio of inhale, exhale and hold must be such, that the practitioner could keep the chosen rhythm for quite a long time with no stress. Of course you can try to do like Indian yoga books say and hold your breath for 40 seconds, but how many respiratory cycles you can do before you want to catch your breath and calm down your heart?

The breath-hold must be a micro-, not a macrostress, it mustn't make you lose your breath and «break» your heart work. Moreover the breath relates to the psyche state, so, if the rhythm of the breath is lost, the psychic state is also dispersed. That's why breath-holds should be harmonically interlaced in the natural breathing rhythm. Note that all these breathings are stressing. If you feel that you cardio-vascular system doesn't cope with it, you are tired, your heart aches, «the hammers» beat in your head, it aches too, all this means that you still have to be careful with these types of breathing.

Doing asanas with breath-holds, **you must know when to stop.** You should not stress neither inhaling, nor exhaling. Your state must be calm. You mustn't strain your jaws, hands, abdominal muscles etc. (as it often happens due to the pathogenic arches).

The breath is hold by the muscles of larynx, so there is actually no need to strain your hands.

Holding your breath after inhaling, you should keep your chest open. Your chest must be open as wide as possible by your inhaling muscles as if you continued inhaling. Then the pressure of lungs on the heart is minimal, and it can beat with the maximum amplitude. Otherwise the heartbeat amplitude shrinks and your heart starts beating faster.

Make sure you keep the same rhythm of breath with holdings for at least one exercise (ideally — during the entire complex). It is important to form a certain well-defined ratio of oxygen and carbonic acid concentration in blood (see the chapter «Types of yoga exercises. Their mechanisms of influence»), which is maintained by a rhythm of breath-holds. The practitioner's task is to achieve a specific state by well-defined ratio of breath-holds. If the time of breath-holds changes, his state «loosens» too.

The capacity to breathe with holds strongly depends on person's vegetative tone. Those who find it difficult to exert themselves (with dominating parasympathetic system) easily do exhaling holds; while those who find it difficult to relax (with dominating sympathetic system) do well inhaling holds. As everywhere, in yoga works the principle of compensation: **you should master the technique, which you do worse.** I.e. people with the ratio of vegetative tone more than 1 (a state when a person is always toned), should learn to make a longer hold on exhale, while those who are constantly relaxed should make a longer hold on exhaling.

You must find your natural and physiological breathing rhythm, in which you can breathe during the entire complex, keeping the same emotional state.

In extreme case you can do an asana on one breathing cycle, entering it and exiting on the first and the one inhalation or exhalation, and to stay in the pose at a breath-hold. Some schools teach this method as the basic. This method is really very effective on conditions that you have a very good health and very clean channels. The last condition is crucial for the following reasons. The energy effect from asana is received, if the energy had time to pass the open channel. The time of passing differs for everyone, depending, as it was already said, on the cleanness of the channel, varying from some minutes to some seconds. If the channel is clogged and the breath-hold is short, it can be just not enough, and asana will become useless.

Besides you should remember that stability of your consciousness in doing the complex (*dharana*) directly depends on keeping one rhythm of breathing during the whole complex. That's why it makes

152

sense to practice this technique only after you're sure that you can do all the planned asanas.

In the morning[1] it makes sense to accent on the inhaling breathing. You can prolong anterior stretching poses to tone yourself up, and in the evening (if you want to avoid a sleepless night, wanting to sleep well) concentrate on the exhale breathing.

Dynamic complexes with breath-holds (by the example of Suria Namaskar)

Suria and Chandra Namaskar as other dynamic complexes can be done with breath-holds. This helps to get the faster effect from the complex, making yoga session faster in general. The principle of accordance of asanas and types of breathing is the same as in static complexes. The chosen breath must enhance the natural effect from asana. The only difference is that exiting one pose we enter another and we do it with the same inhalation or exhalation.

Namaste — rhythmical breathing, hasta uttanasana (pose with risen hands) — inhaling breath, padahastasana — exhaling breath, ashva sanchalanasana (one leg lunge ahead) — inhaling breath, parvatasana (forward set) — inhaling again, Ashtanga Namaskar (zigzagging) — exhaling, «dog» — inhaling, «cat» — exhaling etc. Ideally each pose can be done at one single breath-hold, but only if it's enough to open the needed channel to the full.

---

[1] Here we mean the individual biological morning, which comes for everyone in his time. For example, for «night owls» it comes later than for «morning larks». Before the individual morning it's better not to practice at all.

WORK WITH ENERGY TECHNIQUES

Work with energy through breathing

Practice of work with energy in hatha yoga can be divided into some stages.

At the first level a person works with the energy, which is already present in him, i.e. driving energy from one zone to another. Usually for the first level this energy is enough, because a certain amount of it is held in muscle contractions. In fact we liberate the energy from contractions and muscle blocks, redistributing it more adequately.

If the reader has practiced the described methods with certain regularity, he might have noticed that eventually we get used to them — both physically and energetically. In other words asanas that used to make the heat rise and were causing other physiological sensing of energy moving, don't make the same effect anymore. It is explained not only by adaptation. Those «stocks» of energy, which were kept in muscles, which were used at the beginning are just already redistributed in the body. It becomes more flexible, has less blocks. It's great, but to continue practicing you should come to the next level — getting the energy from outside.

I don't recommend beginners to work with visualisation of energy, because this method is quite difficult and can play some dirty tricks. There are other, simpler, but still very efficient methods to gather energy from the world around you.

The first source of energy you can work with is the air. There is an interesting rule, which was already mentioned: **we gather energy by those parts, by which we «listen» to our physical feelings.** This rule can be easily demonstrated by a simple test. Put your hands one in front of another. «Listen» by your right hand, like the heat is coming from the left hand. After a while your right hand will become warmer and the left one colder. Change the direction of feeling: start «listening» by your left hand for the heat coming from the right one. The right hand will cool and the left start warming. It happens for the said reason: the hand, on which you concentrate, takes the energy — in this case from your other hand. Actually **concentration on sensations is absorbing the etheric energy.**

If we want to take some energy from the air, we must «listen» to the sensation of the air inside or outside ourselves, feel it well.

If we want to gather some energy to a certain chakra, or on the contrary take off some excessive energy from it, we must listen to the feeling of the air at a level of this chakra. If you want to «pump» a channel, you must listen to the feeling of the air at the level of this channel.

This principle is true for all senses. One School has an exercise of eating an orange: you have to eat it very-very slowly, to contemplate it, to sniff it, to touch it, then you slowly cut it, feeling essential oils evaporate, then you eat it, sensing every hue of its taste. As a result a person is full with just one orange, because he absorbs a lot of orange's etheric field. If you eat it quickly, you mostly devour its physical body, ignoring the etheric one.

Every sensory canal relates to a certain chakra and brings energy mostly to it.

The same happens when you work with the etheric energy of the air: breathing without awareness you mostly consume oxygen. If you concentrate on the air passing, you take the *prana* from the air.

There are two basic respiratory exercises you can practice alone or together with the basic complex of exercises to make them more effective. The first one is called *«Breathing up chakras»*. It has for a goal to pump up chakras with the energy of the air.

«Breathing up» chakras

The technique is to pay attention to the air passing each respiratory zone: nasopharynx, larynx, thorax, solar plexus, belly. It's obvious, that each zone relates to a chakra — from Vishuddha to Svadhisthana. Sahasrara and Muladhara aren't nourished by breathing, because sahasrara nourishes by the Cosmic energy and Muladhara — by earth energy. On every chakra it's recommended to do 3-4 breathings.

The better you listen to these sensations, the more energy you take from the air.

Notice that the feeling of the air passing can vary. Some people feel the air *pressing*, its *tickling, coolness* or *warmth*, the *smell*, the *sound* of the moving air. Accenting on various sensations, we take from the air different types of energy. This is the clue to understanding how chakras relate to different sense bodies, which was described in old treatises with no further explanations.

According to Indian sources, Muladhara relates to the smell, Svadhisthana — to the taste, Manipura — to the vision, Anahata to the touch, Vishuddha to the hearing. I suppose that this relation is not absolutely correct, there are some mistakes in texts or in their interpretations. Indeed Muladhara (our physical body) nourishes mostly by food, and in this way more likely corresponds to our **taste** senses. On the other hand, almost for all plants, animals and people, of course, the erotic sense is carried by the smell. That's why I think that Muladhara relates to the taste, and Svadhisthana — to the smell.

Applying this pattern of correspondences on the technique of «taking» the energy from the air, we can say that concentrating on the air's density, we feed our body by the scope of energies close to Muladhara ones, on its smell — we feed Svadhisthana, its temperature (the feeling of warmth) — Manipura, tickling in airways — Anahata, the sound of it passing — Vishuddha.

At the advanced level you should learn to concentrate on the sense, you choose in advance — it trains our sense bodies, our concentration, and bring up to the development of siddhas. On the beginners level it's better to focus on those senses, which are easier to get.

«Breathing up» chakra we can **pump it up** or **cleanse it**. Chakra is pumped up, when the accent is done on the air breathed in. Chakra is cleansed when the accent is done on the air leaving our body on the exhalation. These exercises can be done separately or together.

«Breathing up» channels

Energy from the air can be taken not only at the level of certain chakras, but long all the energy meridians. Especially it's useful to energise active meridians, that's why it makes sense to do this technique together with asanas.

In all anterior-stretching asanas — Bhujangasana, Dhanurasana, Ushtrasana and so on the accent should be done on the air passing through the anterior-middle channel, i.e. you have to «listen» how the air is passing through the anterior part of your lungs.

In posterior-stretching asanas like yoga-mudra, Pashimottanasana, padahastasana, — you should feel the air pass the posterior part of your lungs.

At the advanced level you can coordinate this breathing with the phases of asana. In this case when you enter asana, you can con-

156

centrate on your feelings, then the point of energy gathering will move together with the point separating the stretched part of meridian from the part, still not activated («the stretching point»). When the energy is passing in the static (main) part of asana, the point of gathering is where the energy is naturally passing. For example, in Bhujangasana when the heat passes up the spine, you should concentrate on the air passing the posterior part of your lungs, when you are **exhaling**, if possible, by the same zone, where you feel the heat passing. Such practice teaches us how to move the heat in our body, i.e. to control the energy in our body without doing asanas — just by the conscious effort.

In pivoted asanas like Trikonasana, Arthamatsiendrasana, sarpasana — first of all you must feel the air pass in the stretched lung (feel that you breathe with one lung). And after the energy has passed — in the squeezed one at the exhalation.

«Breathing up»
in pranayamas

Similar clues can be used in pranayamas. For example, when you do anuloma-viloma, breathing in by your right nostril, you should feel the air pass through your right lung as if you where filling by the air only this lung. Exhaling by your left nostril, feel the air leave by the left lung.

In Kapalabhati you should control the air passing in the nasopharynx, front and maxillary sinuses. In Bhastrika you should clearly feel the air in the Manipura zone.

Notice, that problem zones are more difficult to «breathe up». Like in doing asanas unconsciously we try to skip these zones. At the level of depressed or weakened chakras it's more difficult to feel the air pass, although this is what you need to stabilise them. On the contrary, feelings in excited chakras can be too bright, so you need to ignore them.

Work with energy
by visualisation

Visualisation is the most advanced technique of work with energy. **I warn beginners against using this practice in yoga, because visualisation can be easily confused with imagining the energy, which gives no results.** The difference between working with the energy and imagining it, is the same as dining or thinking that you dined.

157

Techniques of «pumping up» in asanas

Asana is a natural energetic outline, so **any work with the energy in asana is applying the outside energy on its natural movement in the body.** Driving the energy by your will against its natural way is in most cases useless or harmful.

No doubt, in entering, staying in the pose and exiting it, the energy moves differently. For example, when you enter Bhujangasana, the anterior channel is opening, and the energy can descend from *the point of entering* (the chin, the third eye or Vishuddha — depending on personal peculiarity) down the point where the stretching arrived. When you are holding the pose, the energy is descending to the lowest point, different in all variations. When it accumulates a lot, sooner or later it goes up the channel located between the anterior and posterior channels, i.e. practically by the spine, closing the energy cycle. That is the main action of Bhujangasana.

In the conscious work you should choose certain energy and put it in the natural passage. In a long stay in asana you can pump up with different energies several times, taking them one by one through the point of entering and driving by the said system of channels. At the first stage you can correlate these energies with your breathing (for example, in Bhujangasana when you breathe in, the energy goes down the front; and when you breathe out, it goes up the back). Later on cleansing your channels you can do without this accordance.

Of course, in asanas not only anterior and posterior middle channels get activated. In asymmetric poses we usually use the channels, located by sides from the central line. If correctly stretched, meridians in the hands and in the legs can also be activated. The scheme of musculotendinous meridians, that can help you to understand activated channels, is given in Appendix.

NOTES

1. The energy can move only in the open, i.e. stretched channel, that's why it makes sense to breathe up in asanas only if they are correctly formed.

2. In a static pose the energy must make a closed loop.

3. Slight variations in asanas' techniques can cause significant changes in energy currents structure (see the chapter «Asanas enhancers»). And vice versa, different variations of asanas are needed to work out and energise different channels.

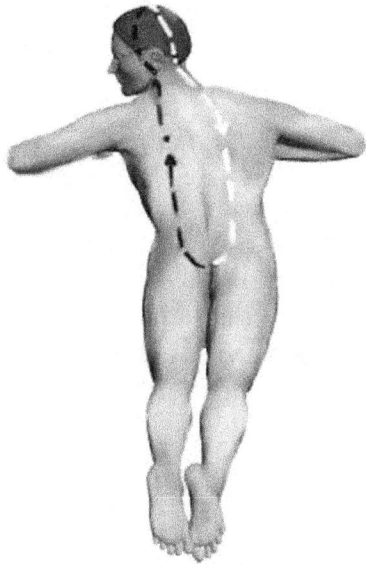

Energy pathway in Sarpasna

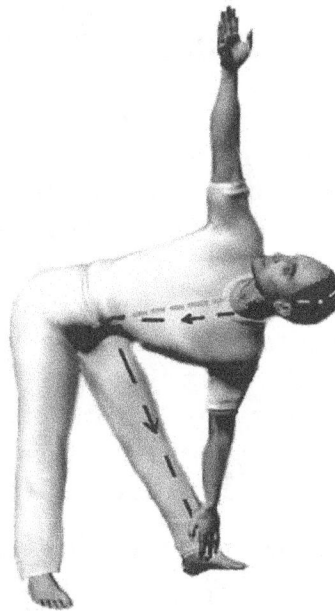

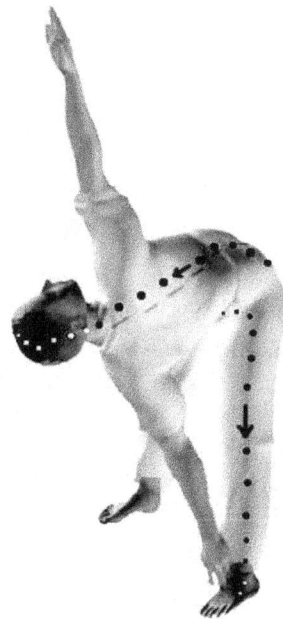

Energy pathway in Trikonasana

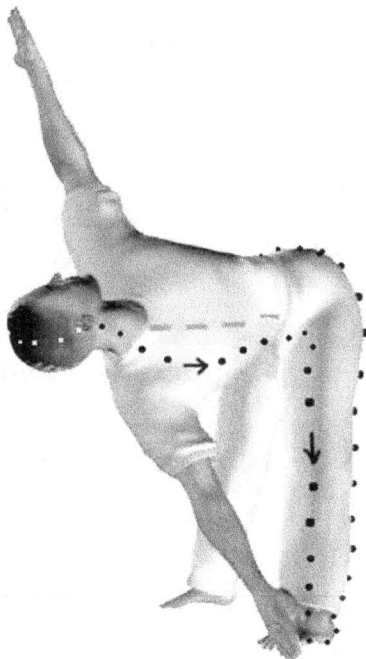

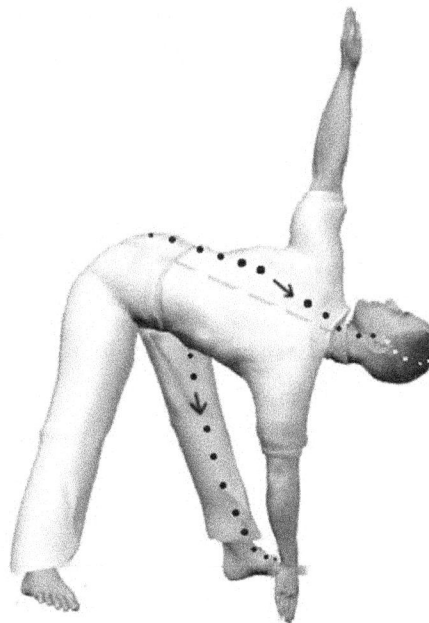

Energy pathway in Trikonasana
(channels in the hands and the outer leg are not shown)

159

«Pumping ups» for men and women

Energy structures of men and women differ, because a man finds easier **to get the energy from above, and a woman — from below. Besides it's easier for a man to take the energy inhaling, and for a woman –exhaling.** Consider that in Bhujangasana and others of that like energy is taken from top down, and in Pashimottanasana and others of that like — from bottom up. Hence asanas can be divided into «masculine» and «feminine», which is perfectly accorded with their effects — relatively toning or calming down, as well as with the believing of Chinese medicine as for the Yin nature of the anterior channel and the Yang — of the posterior, but doing all asanas with no regard to the sex, we should think about differences in «pumping ups».

Variation for men of all pumping ups

The energy is taken from above. Say, you are going to do Bhujangasana, take the energy from above and inhaling drive it down — it's natural, that's the way we do it. Say, you are going to do Pashimottanasna. The energy is still taken from above, but to gather energy before entering the asana we still have one more inhale (when we raise our hands). At this inhale we take the energy from above and drive it by our anterior part of the body down to the coccyx (in yoga-mudra) or down the heels. As a result, exhaling, we start entering asana and we can lift the energy by the opening channel.

Variation for women

In Bhujangasana with the exhalation before entering asana, the energy is taken from below and is driven up the spine till the third eye zone. Inhaling, we enter asana as always, diving the energy down the middle meridian.

In Pashimottanasana the energy is gathered when exhaling, done together with bending ahead, from below immediately to the posterior-middle channel.

Additionally energies are taken from below at the exhalation.

WARNING! Don't be greedy working with energy. Chakras and etheric body have a limited capacity. There is such a state as «overeating»: the energy just doesn't enter anymore. If you pump yourself up efficiently and good, after some pump-ups you can feel oversaturation and laziness. It means, you had enough of it. If you overpump yourself with energies, the effect will be like after a physical overstress. The next morning you'll feel sore and worn out. Sometimes «overeating» makes you feel discoordinated, lazy (not relaxed, but lazy) instead of being sprightly — a normal state after yoga. Find your own energy norm by the experimental method.

ATTENTION! Sometimes in pumping-up or immediately after you can feel heaviness. The main reason is the imperfect physical performance of asanas. The practitioner tries to draw the energy through his clogged or not open channel by his conscious effort. This causes energy tiredness and the wrong distribution of energy in the body, which results in this heaviness.

Another reason can be in the adverse energy in the place of training. For example, if you pump up in the busy public transport, the energy will pass through all auras of passengers, who stand close to you and will bring a lot of energy filth, changing its qualities. Maybe the passengers will rejoice on such cleaning, but will it be healthy for you? A place for doing yoga must be chosen deliberately, taking into account its energy features (not just physical ones), especially the accordance of place's energies with yours. Even in the open air not every place suits every person.

Energy movement in outer etheric

Outer etheric is a part of etheric field, located outside the physical body. Some exercises make the energy move in this part of the etheric. Moreover in some systems, such as tai chi, the main attention is paid to the outer etheric.

Tightening of outer etheric by «raking» movements by hands

To describe and to understand how energy moves in the outer etheric, take the hydrodynamic model. For example, entering Pashimottanasana, there is a compacting of energy in the outer etheric between the hands and ankles due to the energy the practitioner «raked up» by his hands. This excessive energy starts moving the channel, open from the heels. The same happens in padahastasana, Trikonasana etc. Exiting the pose, we smooth the undistributed energy by our hands. Understanding this mechanism, it becomes clear, why hands and arms must be in the right position in asanas, but it's fair to notice that these effects are subtle and not that important at the beginners level.

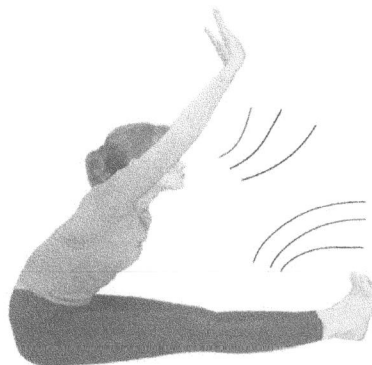

Tightening of energy in the outer etheric

161

How energy «goes out» to the outer etheric in «pumping-ups»

The outer etheric like the inner one has its channels, which get activated, when you do exercises. Usually their filling starts from the centre to peripheries when the inner etheric is filled up. On pictures you see some examples.

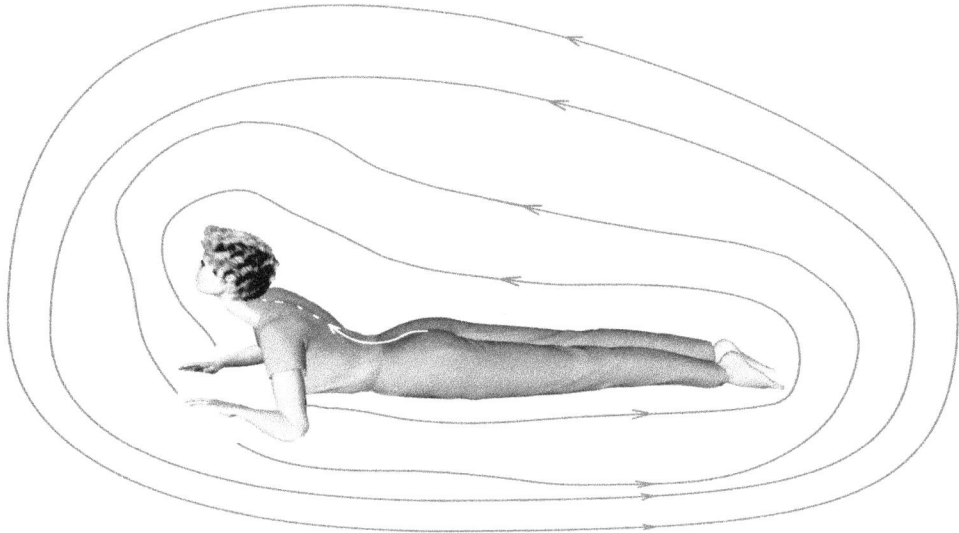

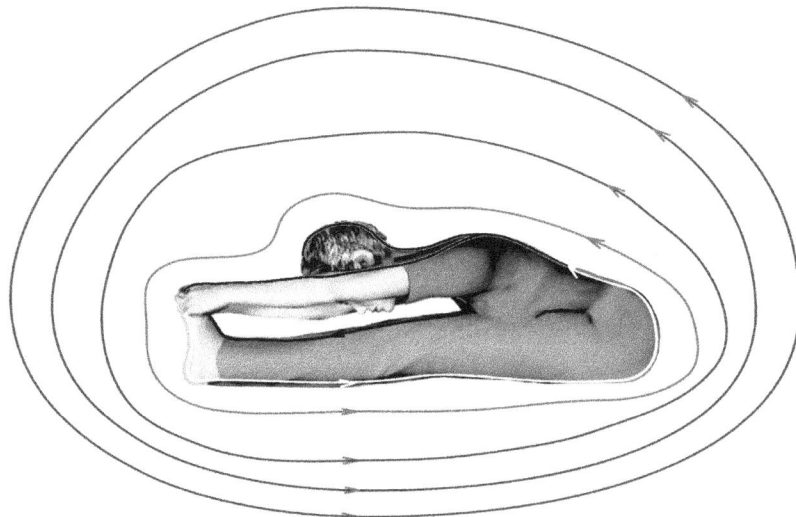

Energy moves in the outer etheric

«Pumping-up» in dynamic complexes

In dynamic complexes energy moves not like in static poses. Speaking about «dynamic complexes» we mean not just Suria and Chandra Namaskar, but other dynamic complexes as well. In a dynamic performance asana doesn't contain a static part, so the energy doesn't make a closed loop. In fact, energy moves only with the strain. In complexes the loop is closed by the next coming asana. In Suria Namaskar hasta uttanasana (pose with risen hands) makes the energy move down the anterior part of the body, and the following pose padahastasana closes the loop, driving the energy up the posterior part. And so on. Each pair of asanas closes the energy loop, enhancing its flow. We, so to say, swirl the energy off, making it stronger. Of course this direction of energy move takes place only if the exercise is done right, first of all, if entering and exiting are done correctly. The anterior stretched asanas must be entered from the head down, and the posterior stretched — from the coccyx (or even heels) up. For example, coming from dog pose to the cat pose is done by lifting the pelvis and not by dropping the head.

Hence pumping up with outer energies should secure this energy movement.

Work with sun mantras

First stage

Repeat a mantra (with no visualisation) in a praying-like elevated state. Repeat and repeat many times until you feel the flow. Sun mantras are pure, so the flow is usually felt as some heat, flushing etc. Like in the physical world there is such thing as inertness, in the astral plane energy doesn't show immediately. To unclog the channel one has to repeat mantra many times. Psyche has to be tuned up. The more you practice, the faster energy shows itself. After a certain practice two-three repetitions of mantra are enough to make energy move, but at the beginning you have to repeat mantra for a long time.

NOTE. There is an effect I call «mantra's breaking up». It can happen when after a while you start saying mantra mechanically and inaccurately, without articulation, swallowing up letters and not noticing these defects. Naturally due to this, the flow disappears or becomes scarcer. To avoid this you must stay aware.

To avoid breaking up mantra Hindu sacrilize the process of reading, doing it in certain rituals. For example, before using mantra you have to rinse your mouth. One could wonder what for — mantras are said mentally — the answer is obvious: to separate the sacred from the profane, to «pump up» the process of reading.

Second stage

When you start feeling the flow, try to see its colour. Even if you fail, you can still visualise the flow coming on you.

How strong the flow is depends on many factors — if there are anomalies on the Sun today, mantras work better of worse (for example, I»ve noticed that sun mantras of Suria Namaskar are especially strong in the top of periods of the Sun activity). Anyway **you can't start visualising the energy until you clearly feel that the flow is really coming, otherwise you'll break up the mantra.**

Mastering of Suria Namaskar mantras is better in the direct sunlight. It better shine directly on the practitioner. It's especially good to start practice with Suria Namaskar mantras in spring, after the vernal equinox, it's the peak of the Sun's getting strong, so mantras work just fine, and you'll feel quicker the effect.

Your forms of work can be different, still once you should try to see the colour of this energy. The colour palette has its advantages. Human's scope of colours is much bigger than the scope of tactical sensations. Mantras of Suria Namaskar are warm and pleasant, but it's very difficult to say which ones are warmer and which ones are colder, although by colour they differ quite a lot.

Note that colours of sun mantras are complicated. They are always underlined by the Sun energy — yellow-orange, but there are two more, interlacing with it — energies of the constellation and of the planet. That's why the mixture is quite complicated.

Emotional aspect of work with sun mantras

Suria Namaskar orientates on Anahata, that's why the feeling of «acceptation» of the Sun helps to get this energy. If a practitioner is closed, he can get **no** energy at all. That's why Suria Namaskar should be done in the elevated and inspired mood.

To make any action arrive, you must fill it with your spirit. Mantras must be filled with your power! In the still state Anahata is closed and the energy doesn't enter your body. All asanas, pranayamas, mudras and mantras should be astrally filled. Then they work.

164

Meditative aspect of work with sun mantras

Unlike most of other mantras, sun mantras, or better say the names of the Sun they contain, can be translated. Each name has a hint on a certain quality a person can possess. Meditation on the essence of this feature and making it come to us, especially together with mantra reading, is the higher level of work with these mantras. Actually meditation on the sense of words is a special kind of spiritual work. Here are translations of 12 main names:

Mitra — friend.

Ravi — shining.

Suria — wonderful light.

Bhanu — diamond.

Bhaga — happiness.

Pushan — empowering.

Hiraniagarbha — golden germ.

Marichia — dawn master.

Aditia — infinity.

Savitar — merciful.

Arka — energy.

Bhaskara — leading to enlightenment.

Maybe these translations don't give fully the essence of these names (it's impossible to translate precisely from one language to another), but it's enough to start practicing. All in all in Vedas and in «Mahabharata» (Araniakaparva) there are 108 names of the Sun.

ASANAS ENHANCERS

The ancient treatises say that the Master of Yoga Siva knew 84 millions of asanas. Nowadays yoga uses about 200 poses, including most sophisticated ones. Where is the rest? How could such a variety exist?

There is one more question: why so different schools give different techniques of the same (by their names) asanas?

The answer to these questions is the following. **Insignificant**, sometimes almost microscopic changes **in the technique of asanas sometimes causes some fundamental changes in their effect, the zone of influence and the direction of their action.** In most cases these changes have to do with the positions of arms and legs, up to fingers and toes. In some poses the limbs become natural weighing material, concentrating our effort in the needed zone, in others specific gestures of fingers activate musculotendinous meridians. These kinds of modifications we'll call pose **enhancers**.

Here are some examples of enhancers, which will help the reader to understand the main idea of this approach in yoga.

Indeed every asana can be slightly modified with insignificant changes in the position of our hands and legs, so that it makes the localised influence on a particular zone. For example, if you do yoga-mudra, the spine zone, which is strained, depends on the position of your hands, playing the role of natural «plummet». So, if you want to work out mainly the middle part of your spine, you should put your hands back, then the main strain will be in the middle spine.

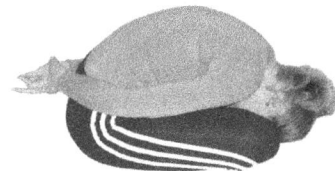

The influence is located mostly in the middle back

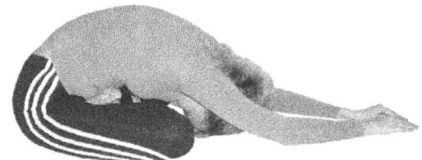

The influence is located mostly in the lower back and the sacral bone

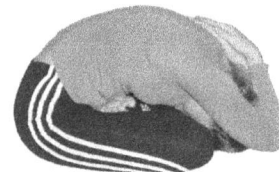

The influence is located mostly in the upper back

166

If you want to work out the lower back, it makes sense to use your arms as a plummet. Then you put your hands before yourself so that they pull you by the shoulders, and the strain goes to the lower back zone. Note that the farther you put your hands, the lower vertebra gets its local influence.

Finally, if you know that your most problem zone is the neck and down the neck, you can put your hands beyond your head. In this case the strain on your neck and the upper spine will be at the maximum.

Sarpasana

This asana can be enhanced, if you draw your leg at the other angle. The farther it's drawn aside, the higher muscles of the back are worked out. It concerns all variations of this asana.

1
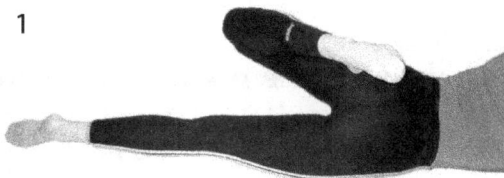

2
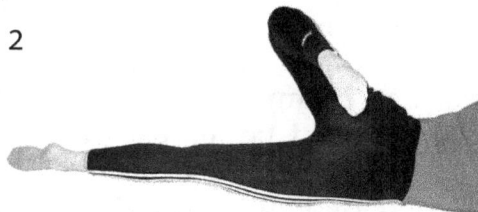

3
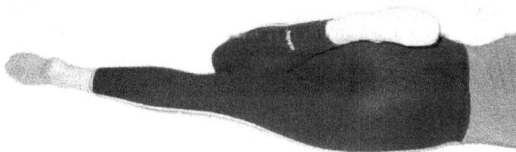

1. The zone of the maximum influence of asana is in Manipura zone left.
2. The zone of the maximum influence of asana is under the left shoulder blade.
3. The zone of the maximum influence of asana is a little up the left buttock.

Pashimottanasana

In Pashimottanasana the role of enhancers is played by your arms. Their position defines, which zone of the spine is worked out (at the same principle as in yoga-mudra).

Arthamatsiendrasana

In Arthamatsiendrasana the role of enhancer is played by your standing leg — the more you pull it to yourself, the lower vertebra are influenced by the asana (with the condition that you are doing it with your back straight and don't take your buttocks off the floor). So, if you have problems with the lower back, you should do Arthamatsiendrasana with your foot almost near your hip, while, if you have problems in the chest zone, you should put the heel almost close to your knee.

167

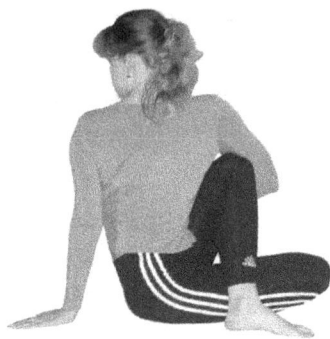

The maximum pivoting in the lower back

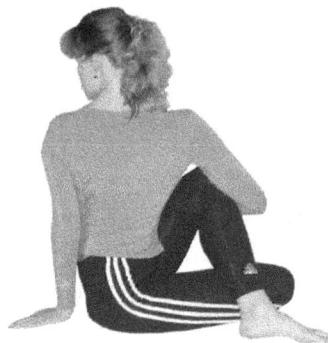

The maximum pivoting in the middle spine

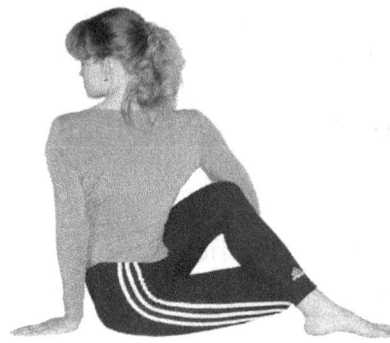

The maximum pivoting in the thorax zone

Marichasana

The enhancer is the angle of the foot of your bended leg. The more you turn it out, the higher in your body feels the pressure from marchiasana. For example, if you want to have an influence on your intestines, the foot should be almost parallel to the other leg. If you want to influence the zone of diaphragm, the spleen (or consequently, if the right leg is bended — on your liver), this foot must be turned out as much as possible.

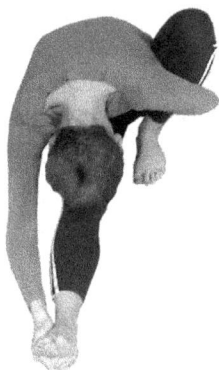

The maximum influence of asana on Svadhisthana zone

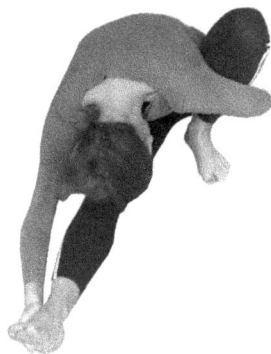

The maximum influence of asana on Manipura zone

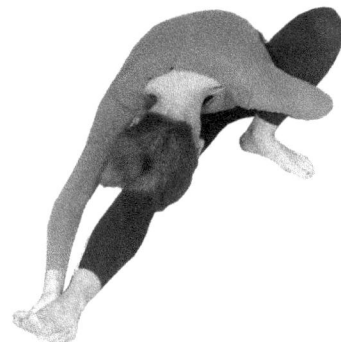

The maximum influence of asana on Anahata zone

Trikonasana

The enhancers in this pose are angles between your legs and your feet.

Dhanurasana

The enhancers in dhanurasana are similar to those in Ushtrasana.

168

Ushtrasana

The enhancer in Ushtrasana is the angle between the knees. The more they are apart, the lower chakras get worked out.

The maximum influence on Anahata

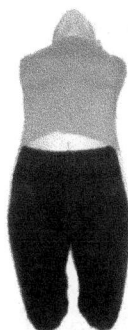

The maximum influence on Svadhisthana

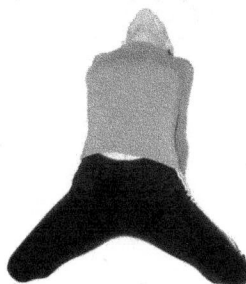

Arthasalabhasana

The enhancer in this asana is the angle of drawing your leg aside. The more it's stretched aside, the higher muscles of the spine are influenced.

NOTE. The angle between your legs is the enhancer, not only because your weight is redistributed, but also because different musculotendinous meridians get involved (see Appendix 2).

Sirshasana

The enhancer in Sirshasana is the angle between your elbows. The wider they are, the less your bearing area is, the more difficult it is to keep balance, and the lower chakras get involved.

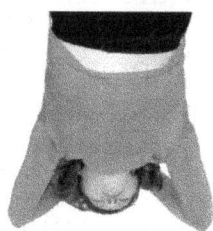

The maximum influence on Anahata zone

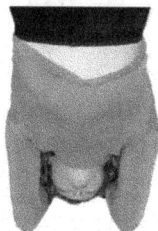

The maximum influence on Vishuddha zone

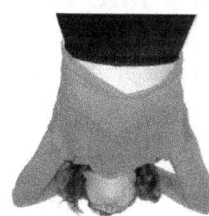

The maximum influence on Muladhara zone

Almost every asana has its enhancers. Guided by your understanding of their principles, you can adjust asanas and yoga complexes in the way that they work out your most problem zones.

Yoga is not a dogmatic studying, but a set of principles and instruments, which every practitioner can and should use creatively to achieve his own goals and tasks.

MEDITATIONS

As you know, meditation is one of the oldest methods of influence on one's psyche. However, being the powerful instrument of the spiritual development, meditation can become a powerful tool of self-destruction. The many thousand year veil of secrecy on the one hand and the enthusiastic smatterer's approach on the other have caused the fact that only one percent of those who practice meditative techniques really achieve some positive changes in their psyche. The main reason is the absence of system approach to meditations. Besides the most important thing is forgotten: **meditation is an instrument, not the goal of spiritual development.** To use an instrument, you must know what it's for, how to apply it and you must have a clear plan of what you want to do. The last point is what most inexperienced practitioners miss. They often use meditation like an unknown pill, without any prescription, just because they know, that drugs cure, but they ignore that every drug has its specific influence on our body.

It's fare to notice that there were and there still are schools that use a scientific approach to meditative practices. For example, coming to a Tibetan monastery, a student was given a task to practice one of the 108 classic meditations — the one his teacher thought his psyche needed the most. The same approach is used in serious schools of yoga.

In this chapter we'll take a look at the principle of choosing meditations and at some meditative techniques, which can be useful at the beginners' level of yoga.

Psychological aspects of meditation

From the psychological point of view there can be defined five main directions of inside work with one's own psyche.

1. Actualisation of psychic's processes.
2. Development of consciousness and of self-consciousness.
3. Cleansing of subconsciousness.
4. Deprogramming of super-consciousness.
5. Achieving the inner integrity.

Let's take a more detailed look at every direction and study its origins.

Actualisation of psychic's processes

A significant volume of information, taken by our senses, isn't fixed in our consciousness. We look and don't see, we listen and don't hear, eat and don't taste. The main reason for it is that the most of time our consciousness isn't «here and now», instead it's busy solving different problems, remembering images of the past and telling what wasn't said in time. The same was with our emotions, feelings and strivings, which aren't always conscious, but still they influence our life, underlying our actions and attitude. According to Gestalt all this results in the fact that a person has less free energy, which means he is less adaptive to life situations. To solve this problem we can practice the «here and now» state — on the level of our senses, emotions and feelings.

The notion of the importance of actualisation of psychic processes appeared already in ancient systems of psycho-practices. A lot of attention was paid to it by tantra. Many of 112 meditations described in «Vijniana Bhairava Tantra» are dedicated to actualisation.

«Open the door to your senses. Feel even the ant creep. Then THIS will come».
Vijniana Bhairava Tantra

Actualisation was an important part of Zen. We know a parable about a Zen master, who became a student again, because he forgot on which side of his umbrella he left his sandals — he realised that did it mechanically.

Among contemporary esoteric schools the biggest attention to actualisation was paid by G. Gurdgieff, who broached the subject of actualisation even before F. Perls and Osho. One of his most impressing techniques is probably the «Stop», which is done like this: a group of students do their everyday work and in the most unexpected moment get the order to freeze. At the same moment they must stop, being conscious of the position the order caught them in. In his «Orange book» Osho describes the following actualisation techniques: smoking meditation, desautomatisation and others. The most complete studying the actualisation of psychic processes got in Gestalt-psychology of F. Perls, which quite soon turned from a psychotherapeutic system into a semiesoteric school. The main importance of these psycho-techniques is in the fact that they don't only widen the consciousness by actualisation, but also in the smoothest way teach people to reflect, which is crucial for the work at further levels.

Development of consciousness and of self-consciousness

Followers of the contemporary esoteric systems especially emphasize the crystallisation of consciousness and the development of self-consciousness. This apparently correlates with the appearance of existentialism and the respective discourses. It's also possible that the respective psychopractices became relevant under the influence of corresponding philosophic ideas. For example, the notion of «consciousness crystallisation» was introduced to the occult tradition by Gurdjieff. By this he meant forming a stable inside world in a person. The famous researcher of his works professor A. Rovner noticed that some of these ideas appeared under the influence of Nietzsche. An extremely important, if not the central role, the consciousness played in the study of D. Krisnamurti. There are many efficient techniques of crystallization of consciousness in works of C. Castaneda.

Among techniques proposed by C. Castaneda first of all is significant the «Thinking about Death» technique. According to it you must be constantly aware, that every moment of our life, including the present, can be the last one, because «death is always standing behind your left shoulder». The effect of this meditation implies that the last moment of life, when there is already no future and the past loses its value, a person would certainly want to live fully, i.e. consciously. This technique isn't really new. Almost the same technique was described in Samurai codex Bushido. However the philosophic description of similar techniques was given by Heidegger and Sartre. Utterly efficient for crystallization of consciousness are exercises of stalking, proposed by Castaneda — the art of a conscious action — like «Transformation» or «Transformation in woman» etc. The effect from these techniques comes from the fact, that, playing an unusual role, a person is obliged to keep his consciousness continuously alert. Choosing a new unusual role, better completely opposite to all past experience, at a good concourse of circumstances helps to feel inside one's own Being.

172

Speaking about Gurdjieff's system, we'll notice first of all the «Stop» technique, described above. The effect of crystallization of consciousness arrives thanks to the actualisation, related to this process.

Among meditations of Osho, which have the same goal, it's worth to mention «Are you here», «Become a cosmonaut of your inside space», «Don't try to fool yourself», described in his «Orange book» and so on.

Note that some meditations of classical esoteric systems were also favouring the crystallization of consciousness. Thus in yoga there was a technique «Observation of fire or of the light between eyebrows».

In this meditation one had to feel the light radiate from inside, so that the consciousness would be its source, not just an external observer. The already studied technique «Growing the spiritual child» is a variation of consciousness crystallization, practiced in Taoist yoga.

Cleansing of subconsciousness

The notion of «subconsciousness cleansing», i.e. reacting the suppressed feelings and emotions, causing neurotic tension, also appeared thanks to the ideas of psychoanalysis. Although these techniques of cleansing were used by mankind for all the times. They are so numerous, but can be divided into two categories:

Analytical — are based on realizing unconscious objects and using them together with their secondary manifestations (dreams, emotional tensions etc.). To practice them one must already have quite a wide consciousness (a solid ego, by psychoanalytic) and a good capacity of reflection. The most part of analytical methods have roots in different schools of psychoanalysis, but are actually similar to the Buddhist vipassana, described above.

Catharsis — are based on the direct reacting of bothering feelings and emotions, with no need to realize them. These are for example, the cry therapy, breathworks like rebirthing, holotropic breathwork and others.

Cleansing of subconsciousness is an important step in self-transformation not only because it helps to diminish neurosis, typical to a modern person, but also because it liberates psychic energy, needed for deeper internal work. Osho proposed quite a wide range of techniques, being so different, that anyone could choose the meditation that could liberate him from a certain kind of non-realised emotions. Actually Osho has redone on the modern level the Buddhist practice of personal selection of meditation. Here are some techniques from his «Orange book».

173

«Dynamic meditation» — a real find of Osho. An efficient meditation of the catharsis type.

«Laughing meditation» — helps to liberate oneself from non-realised emotional energies and is a practice of artificial laugh during a certain time. The task is to achieve a moment, when the laugh would go naturally, with no more need to force it.

«Beating of the pillow» — helps to let go the suppressed aggression.

«Breathe like a dog» — catharsis meditation, using the power of breath. Favours to react the aggression.

«Nataraja meditation» — catharsis meditation helping to react the energy, underlying hurry and bustling.

«Jolting» — a catharsis meditation, setting free the muscles, liberating unconscious desires.

«Peering at the mirror» — an effective meditation, helping to actualise unconscious fears.

«Come into your fear» — the effect is similar to the previous meditation.

Typical for meditations, proposed by Osho, is that almost all of them provoke catharsis.

In Castaneda system there is a curious technique called «Wiping off the personal history» or «Returning the lost energy», which from the psychological point of view can be interpreted as the one aiming to cleanse the subconsciousness. The most full description of it is given in the «Sorcerer's crossing» by Taisha Abelar. It implies «returning back the energy lost in past situations and in liberation of energies received in such situations from others».

Transpersonal physiotherapy also has some very efficient methods of cleansing the subconsciousness. Among them we can mention holotropic breathwork, one-way, rebirthing, based on catharsis power of breathing, psychoanalytical techniques, body-oriented psychotherapy and many others. Psychotherapeutic techniques unlike those of yoga imply the presence of a therapist, correcting patient's actions, which significantly increases their therapeutic effect (of course, if the therapist is a highly professional specialist). In general we can note that psychotherapy became a bridge to esoterism for the European culture.

Deprogramming of super-consciousness

Deprogramming of super-consciousness is the liberation from stereotypes, directives and complexes, imposed in childhood. It is also viewed by the followers of contemporary esoteric systems as an element of self-work.

Already Freud noted the fact that components of super-consciousness are the source of the majority of psychological problems. The creator of transact analysis E. Berne was the first to describe in details the role of parents' programming in human's life, but he proposed no efficient techniques of liberation from these programs. Nevertheless such techniques as reframing (described below) appeared later, thanks to the methods of Erickson's hypnosis, Neuro-linguistic programming, but most of them don't deprogram the super-consciousness, but reprogram it, i.e. replace some programs by others, more efficient for a person. Also note that the possibility itself to deprogram and reprogram the super-consciousness results in creating new philosophic and ethic questions of whether one value system (with its programs) is better than another. The most attention to deprogramming is paid by the followers of «rebel» Zen and of the similar systems. It's interesting to notice that the transact analysis itself together with other systems, practicing inside deprogramming, appeared in the second half of XX century, when the society was eagerly reviewing its old values, actually deprogramming its collective superconsciousness». On the other hand it was the time when the public first learned about ideas and practical results of cybernetics, which provoked the wish to describe human's psyche in the same terms. «The consciousness and the body are parts of the same cybernetic machine». The cybernetic system appeals by its seeming simplicity. We can accept it or not, but we can't deny that in desidentification with one's behaviour patterns it's more helpful than all philosophic arguments of humanitarian psychological schools.

Let's take a look at some techniques of inside deprogramming, used in different esoteric systems.

«Inside hunting» is a technique given by C. Castaneda. It implies the conscious «tracing down» of your stereotypic acts, that are obstacles to your development, and their eventual removal. The same goals have exercises like «Changing of one's appearance», «Breaking the regime», Destructuralisation of ego», described by the same author.

«Reframing», a technique used in NLP, clearly has mystic roots. It is based on searching for situations, where the superconscious program wasn't correct and following it in an absurd way. Realizing this situation, a person can get a catharsis discharge of the program.

Achieving inner integrity

The highest phase of self-transformation in most of occult systems is **the achieving of inner integrity**, which presumes the synthesis of various parts of human's psyche (subpersonalities). In fact the detection of non-integrity of human's personality is one of the most curious discoveries, done almost at the same time by mystics and psychologists. The category of **subpersonality** itself, broadly used in Gestalt-psychology, psychosynthesis and later appeared in role theory of Mead, was first introduced by Gurdjieff, although the existence of subpersonalities was already described by Patanjali.

4.4. Created minds (I suppose he speaks about subpersonalities) arise from egoism alone.

4.5. There being difference of interest, one mind is the director of many minds.

4.6. Of these, the mind born of concentrated insight is free from the impressions (he is speaking about forming the stable basic personality on the base of Inside Observer)

Yoga-Sutra

Subpersonalities are stable structures, partly having consciousness, emotions, desires and other features, so to say expressing different facets of human's personality. Gurdjieff was comparing human's psyche with the battlefield where different parts fight for control over human's behaviour. If there is no «Master», i.e. person's real «I», which can be crystallized from the contains of his psyche by a hard inside work, this fight never ends. It can be easily seen when a person is doubting, trying to decide between two alternatives. These doubts are in fact the fight of his two or more subpersonalities, having different opinions. Depending on which one will win, a person takes this or another decision. Another clear example of subpersonalities is the inside dialogue — a talk of subpersonalities. Gurdjieff didn't know about the ideas of cybernetics, so he described this process in mechanic terms — although in his description we can easily see that human's psyche can be programmed. The main task of his system can be defined by the following: «A person must stop being a machine and try to become a Human». From this task he developed different precise techniques of work with subpersonalities.

In the work with subpersonalities we can define two goals. **A minimum task is to achieve a coherent state of psyche,** i.e. a state when there is no fight between different subpersonalities — they all cooperate for the same goal. For this we can use various techniques of the inside treaties, we can use the six-step model of the inside treaty proposed by NLP. The more complicated task is to integrate all subpersonalities, i.e. to achieve an integral state of consciousness. A person who achieved this state can be himself in any situation, having no need — neither inside, nor outside, — to play any roles. Techniques that help to achieve this state are described in works of Roberto Assaggioli and his followers (for example, D. Rainwater). Some techniques were described by Osho, including meditations «Funny faces» and «Looking in the mirror» can be used to actualise your subpersonalities.

In classical esoteric systems there also are methods that can be interpreted as those of synthesising subpersonalities to achieve the inside integrity. First of all it's the Tibetan method of merging with *idams*. From the psychological point of view idams can be interpreted as personifications of different parts of human psyche, especially since in

176

Tibetan yoga tradition idams are openly declared «the fruit of the mind». In this case the merging with idams can be viewed as a technique of a successive symbolic actualisation of subpersonalities, relating to different layers of the unconscious, with the following synthesising them. Tibetan sources consider that these practices should be done with cautious, because, if a subpersonality is weaker by its energy potential than the consciousness, the later can be dissolved in the subpersonality. That's why Tibetan teachers give their pupils a well-defined sequence of idams for meditation.

Work with subtle bodies

As it was said in the chapter «Types of yoga exercises and their mechanisms of influence» a meditation can be seen not only from psychological, but also from the energy point of view. In this case **meditation is an exercise for the astral body** (rarer for the mental body, such meditations are scarce). Goals of these exercises include:

1. Involving in the energy circulation the idle part of the astral plane. This goal is the same as the previously discussed widening of the consciousness and cleansing of subconsciousness.
2. Searching for individual clues to work with energy.
3. Manipulation with chakras' fields and with «energy bearing». Let's take a detailed look at it.

There are two extreme states of astral field of every chakra: **the extreme tightening** and **the extreme widening** of the field.

For example, the state of extreme tightening in Anahata is achieved by a meditation of «disidentifying oneself with emotional states of others». At the energy level the practitioner «throws away» from his field all the states that, despite being in his field, are not his own, being something, he caught from outside: irritation, hurry, emotions of others etc. Tightening of Ajna is a disidentification with all the roles we play, getting rid of depersonification states. The Manipura tightening makes you ready for the situation and able to count just on yourself, the Svadhisthana — a clear feeling of your desires etc.

The contrary state — Anahata's widening is feeling the state of others — the empathy. The extreme widening of Anahata is a state when you can feel the emotional state of any person (any place or egregor) as your own. Widening of the field of upper chakras is creativity, widening of Ajna is the capacity to read «the signs of the world», to get information from different egregors; of Vishuddha — the capacity to rely on other's point of view like on your own, of Manipura — using situations and resources of the world etc.

Widened states are very important, because **only in the widen state chakras receive energy**. A person, unable to widen the field of some chakras (which means they are rigid), sooner or later gets them empty.

One can't constantly live in such extreme states — they can only be achieved in meditation.

The essence of practicing wide-tightened states is to train oneself to get extreme states and to widen the attainable scope of states in every chakra. Such emotional-psychological flexibility helps to find and to form a state of field, optimal for a current life situation.

Practice of meditation is building an hierarchy of states from the extreme tightening to extreme widening of the astral field as well as finding one's own balanced state, and training oneself to take an adequate state in every situation.

In addition to widening and tightening of fields, every chakra can have a so called «energy bearing» — a specific state, a configuration of the field, which has a certain influence on others. Some energy bearings are pathogenic, like the ones «provoking» people on the negative attitude to you. An example of such energy bearing can be a state «you want to fight with me?» viewed by people like a challenge and sooner or later leading to a conflict. There are also useful energy bearings, such as the state of «the boss», when a person is viewed like someone important not only by his employees, but even by those who don't know him personally. Conventionally energy bearings can be divided into giving, taking and neutral. The last ones make it possible to stay unnoticed.

Every posture taken consciously is a siddha. The task of yoga on the advanced levels (beyond the subject of this book), is forming of capacities to achieve as wide repertory of energy bearings as possible.

Vows

The practice of meditations can be significantly enhanced by the practice of *vows*. Almost in all esoteric traditions vows were the strongest instrument of psychological self-influence, used almost in all cultures. However the greatest development this practice got in the Indian tradition. Mahabharata and other mythological sources are rich in describing huge spiritual achievements, thanks to vows. In the Christian tradition this practice was significantly primitivised, that's why to our time came the belief that vows aim at the development of the will. However in the Eastern tradition vows are used for much deeper inside work. By their action, vows can be divided into two groups.

178

Vows, **limiting** certain functions of a person, like *brahmacharia*[1] (refusal from the sex life), the vow of silence, fasting and so on. Limiting one of his natural functions, a person accumulates and enhances a certain type of inner energy, which helps to actualise it and then to put under the conscious control.

«As soon as you get an impulse to do something, stop».

Vidzhniana Bahirava Tantra

Vows, **positively defining** a person's form of behaviour, helps to accumulate energy, to actualise inside problems and to solve them. The longer it lasts, the deeper inside problems get disclosed.

Work with mental body. Djnana yoga

Our mental body contains the following.

1. Person's life position is the deep disposition to oneself and the world around, a person's individual matrix, a prism, through which he is looking at the world. It contains an emotional aspect and is a bridge between the astral and mental bodies. Usually life position is not realised, though it's possible and even not very difficult to do. In most cases the life position can be described by a short metaphor, like four life positions by Berne: I'm OK—You're OK; I'm not OK—You're OK; I'm OK—You're not OK; I'm not OK—You're not OK.

The life position, conscious or not, is going through the whole person's life, significantly predetermining it. An unfavourable, non-harmonic life position can significantly worsen the quality of life and to influence person's self-realisation in social and spiritual spheres, and even on his health. That's why the task to actualise the life position and to correct it, if needed, is so important.

The structural contain of the life position is the emotional filling of notions. Take a vitally important notion, which is a mental structure itself, and concentrate on it. You'll finds out that many notions contain an emotional element. Negative emotions about some notions make it harder to contact with the respective object in the physical plane. For example, the negative filling of the category «society» makes a person socially less adaptive, and the one of the category «money» makes him poor.

---

[1] This definition is not exact, but widely known, for more details see chapter «Yoga and sex».

2. Person's worldview is a more complicated construction. It's hard to be expressed by a simple metaphor. Greatest philosophers were writing volumes, trying to describe their worldview, but for most of people their worldview is unconscious and often contradictory. In this case sooner or later these oppositions are realised in the physical plane.

The base for every worldview is person's individual values — certain objects, states and thesis, having for him an unconditional importance. Values can be conscious and unconscious. If they are unconscious, there can be a problem: a person who starts living in a system of values, different from his own, imposed from outside (for example, by a subculture in which he found himself), starts breaking down. Not in metaphoric, but in the direct sense. That's why actualisation of one's values and worldview is not a funny game, but a vital necessity on the way of spiritual development.

From the worldview logically come **senses**. The worldview always includes a sense-forming, value aspect, otherwise it's not a worldview, but a «knowledge about..».. Senses like values aren't always realised by a person. There can also be (and even quite often) a **pseudo-worldview:** what a person thinks is his worldview, doesn't really determine his life, being just a system of rationalisation, directed to explain personal problems and the unwillingness to solve them. Analysing life of the greatest thinkers of the past, we can see that they became «great», exactly because they succeeded in reflection and in reconstruction of their own worldview as well as in living according to it, i.e. in making it real.

An important task of djana yoga is to achieve a congruency of one's life and worldview.

3. Mode of thinking. An inner logic, which can differ from the common «Aristotle's» logic.

In last decades the science has proved, that a non-Aristotle's logics can exist, like the alternative geometry that differs from the common Euclid geometry. The person's way of thinking can be not harmonic inside and be realised as some psychological and eventually physical problems. By the way, some researches prove that mentally ill patients have their own specific logic.

The work with mental body is based on **the reflection of thinking,** i.e. the capacity to see internal contradictions in one's thinking, as well as to track down the methodology of thinking, it's style and the style of thinking of others, to adjust one's thinking according to a certain task.

Other techniques of djana-yoga are beyond the tasks of this book.

180

YOGATHERAPY. SOME PRINCIPLES OF BUILDING THERAPEUTIC COMPLEXES

WARNING! This chapter is written for instructors, healers and advanced practitioners. If you don't understand something, never build your own therapeutic complexes — consult a specialist.

Most of the yoga books say about therapeutic effect from asanas, enlisting organs, which these poses influence and treat. However, if it's easy to agree with the «influence», which is also easy to check — it's enough to take this pose and to see what you feel; it's more complicated with asana's treating effect. Indeed every organ can have absolutely different diseases with completely different reasons and needing absolutely different approaches to the treatment. That's why such an approach is not professional. Yoga exercises are really very strong medicaments, but like pills, they need to be used right, moreover, being taken wrong, they can become harmful. To understand principles of yoga-therapy let's take a look at the methodology, underlining it.

Counterbalancing of branches of autonomic nervous system (ANS)

According to contemporary science a normal functioning of human's body is provided by his autonomic (vegetative) nervous system, which contains the sympathetic and parasympathetic branches. Curiously this notion have a lot in common with the Indo-Tibetan medicine, which acknowledged two basic principles of body's functions: «heat» and «cold».

It's very rare to see a person with balanced branches of ANS. Usually this balance is shifted to either side.

If it is disbalanced significantly without compensation, there can be symptoms of illness and functional disorders. Sympatics can have such diseases as hypertension, arteriosclerosis and coronary disease. Parasympatics can typically have stomach and duodenum ulcers, bronchial asthma etc.

The contemporary medicine put the outward signs into special tables (table of Wein).

It's also possible to tell the ergo- and trophotropic activity by the test of Luscher, often used in psychology.

Sympatics are recommended to do bending asanas like Pashimottanasana and yoga-mudra. Exercises should be done with no hurry, with Svadhisthana or Anahata set-up with the long fixation in the posture. It's good to begin with such asanas as shavasana. Besides sympatics are indicated to breathe through the left nostril (Chandra bhedana) and to do Suria Namaskar complex.

To treat disorders related to the excessive parasympathetic activity, the best are anterior arching poses like Bhujangasana[1]. Exercises should be done in the active pace. It's good to practice Suria Namaskar with Manipura set-up, as well as small pranayamas and kumbhaka. Sympathetic system is also toned by Suria bhedana (breathing through the right nostril).

The principles of taking into account the factor of dominating ANS branch in building therapeutic complexes are in more detail discussed in the article of Sergey Agapkin «Building individual practice according to principles of Indo-Tibetan medicine».

However the given scheme of dividing people into sympatics and parasympatics is not unconditional. It's noticed that sometimes a person can have signs of both columns of Wein's table, i.e. one person can have signs of activated branches of both sympathetic and parasympathetic systems. This observation comes along with the yogic concept of depressed and excited chakras, as the energy reason of disease. Because chakras correspond the knots of ANS, **it's possible to have one chakra (and the respective ANS branch) depressed and another — excited.**

---

[1]   According to research of the author using colour tests of Luscher, practice of Bhujangasana increases the ration of vegetative tone in 1.5 times.

Evaluation of initial vegetative tone by Wein

Sign	Sympathicotomy (predominance of sympatics)	Vagotonia (predominance of parasympatics)
Complexion	Pale	Reddish
Vascular pattern	Not pronounced	Marble-like, acrocyanosis
Sebaceousness of skin	Reduced	High, acne
Sweating	Reduced	High, hyperhidrosis
Dermographism	Rose, white	Red, prominent
Chill	Absent	Typical
Fever within infections	Bias towards hypothermia	Usually not big, bias towards mild pyrexia
Portability of stuffy spaces	Satisfactory	Bad
Syncope	Rare	Typical
Dizziness, vestibulopathy	Not typical	Typical
Appetite	High	Can be reduced
Body mass	Bias towards thinness	Possible bias towards obesity
Heartbeat	Bias towards tachycadria	Bias towards bradycardia
Arteriotony	Bias towards high	Bias towards low
Cardialgy	Possible	Often, with no apparent reason
Lacking of air, «sighing»	Not typical	Typical
Bias towards nausea, vomiting, pain in the stomach	Not typical	Possible
Pain in legs by the end of the day, at night	Not typical	Can be
Headaches	Can be mostly with emotional tension	Often after overstrain, migraine-like
Sleep	Anxious	Deep, long lasting

Human energy anomalies as a reason of disease

Excited and depressed chakra

According to a yoga concept, human's state is determined by his subtle bodies and planes, first of all, etheric and astral, which are projected on the physical body. The reason why these bodies become distorted is the breaking of Natural laws, primarily negative energy connections with other people, called «tails». An example of such connection can be some hurt feelings of one person by another, the feeling of guiltiness or responsibility, obsession or excessive attachment.

«Tails» can be conventionally divided into taking ones, when the energy is leaving us, and giving ones — when the energy is coming to us. The same tail is giving to one person and taking for another. Long-lasting energy inflow or outflow first distorts person's aura, playing the role of a buffer (when so called «holes», «bumps» and «dents» appear), and then his inside energy structure. With the long-lasting outflow from a chakra, where the tail is located, chakra becomes depressed, and after a long inflow — excited. At the same time chakra's localisation slightly changes. The experience has shown that an **excited chakra shifts forward,** to the anterior part of the body; **while the depressed one moved back.**

By person's posture it's easy to see his customary excited and depressed chakras. There is a general principle: spine's posture repeats the chakral structure. **At the level of excited chakra person's vertebra moves slightly forward, and he starts arching. At the level of depressed chakra a person starts stooping.**

Unlike the previously described situation with field's looseness, when a person can move by an area deliberately, a person with a depressed chakra is constantly stooping in this area. Even when he is asked to stand straight, he can't do it, because his inner criteria of «straightness» differ from the apparent view. For example, if a person has a constantly depressed Anahata, he's stooping in the heart zone. According to the depressed zone, he can stoop in his upper, middle or lower Anahata.

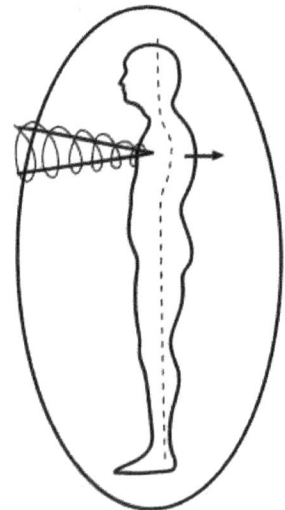

Breaching in the etheric body

184

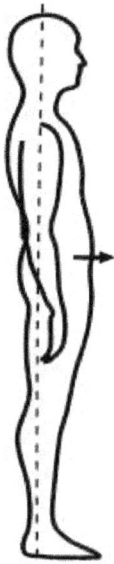

Posture of a person with an excited Svadhisthana

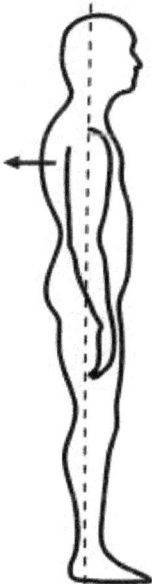

Posture of a person with a depressed Anahata

If a person has a constantly depressed Manipura, he always tries to sit down, «tucking in» his belly, the zone retires and closes (though it's not called «stooping»). If a person has a depressed Vishuddha, he usually hides it in the shoulders, lifting them and bows his head. If Vishuddha is excited, a person looks «through his nostrils» — his head is always slightly dropped back.

If a person has an excited Ajna, he walks like an ostrich — a head always before his body. If Ajna is depressed, the head is slightly dropped back. If Svadhisthana is depressed a person hides this zone, if excited — sticks it out. It's easy to understand why it happens on energy level.

For example, let's take the heart chakra. If Anahata is depressed, it shifts back, taking along human's etheric body. It forms a hole, unnatural to a human. A person tries to smooth his etheric as he can — by stooping at the respective angle. A person stoops, the edges of the hole got closer, the density of etheric is relatively equal — forward and back. The same happens when chakra is excited. Chakra shifts forward, where appears a bump, while at the back — a dent. By straightening his shoulders he compensates them.

What are the breaches causing chakra depression? **Most often chakra becomes depressed, when a person spends too much energy from this chakra.** There can be several ways of such overspending.

The first way of energy loss is due to **hypertrophic emanation.** Mostly chakra ends up in this phase after an overexcitation. For example, a person has breaches on Ajna — he constantly tries to persuade others in his worldview, others resist as they can, but he argues, presses them down, proves logically, people continue resisting, but he «explains them the truth» and so on. In the end either his opponents give up, or get rid of him — in both cases he loses his energy. The state of overexcitation demands high excitation of chakra, when the person keeps this state. A person with the excited Ajna is almost impossible to persuade. Any attempt to communicate with him at this chakra will end with him giving you a bunch of examples; and even if you succeed in making some more logical arguments, he will never listen to you.

185

After a year or two (everyone has his time) chakra becomes constantly depressed, i.e. the person exhausted himself. If a person has a depressed Ajna, he finds it very difficult to concentrate on something — his thoughts are bouncing from one subject to another, hardly fix on something precise, and he gets easily obsessed by changing ideas, having a state of general misbalance.

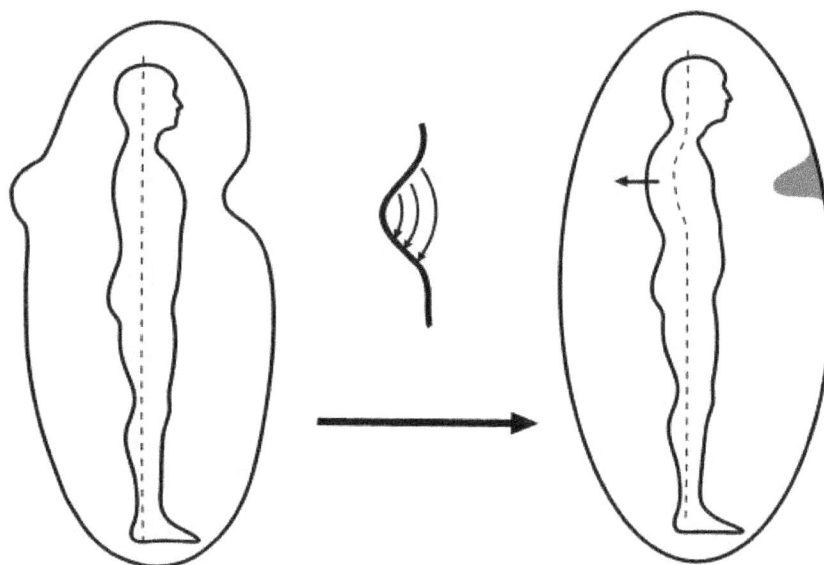

Mechanism of Anahata's depression with the field breached

A second way of losing energy is **wasting it by tails.** If chakra has many taking tails, energy is leaving it unconscious to its owner. It looks as if a debtor pays the interest automatically, at the moment, when money arrive to the bank — a person doesn't even see it. By the way, the one, who feels guilty, really pays by his Manipura energy.

Let's briefly describe states, related to dysfunctions of other chakras.

Depression of Vishuddha can be defined as **inexpressiveness.** A person doesn't express himself, inside he can be very interesting with interesting thoughts, interesting inner life, but all this doesn't find its way out. In the state of excited Vishuddha a person strived to say something even if he has nothing to say.

The state of **depressed Anahata** is **the emotional depression,** when a person isn't disposed to emotional feelings and can hardly feel joy etc. On the contrary, if one's Anahata is excited, he has high emotionality, a state, when a person gets high from his own emotions. Eventually it can end with burning out Anahata.

186

A person with **a depressed Manipura** is a perfect employee, who must have his Manipura depressed to follow quickly directives — on the energy of his boss. With an excited Manipura a person is an eternal squabbler.

The state of **depressed Svadhisthana** is a state of sexual underdevelopment, lowered sexuality, boredom. The state of excited Svadhisthana appears after long holding of the sexual desire.

It's difficult to say about Muladhara, as it doesn't move forward or back, but still it can be breached.

Actually other ways of chakra's excitation are also possible — when it gets excited not because its owner overrealizes himself on it, but because he gathered too much energy on it by this or another method. For example, having a hypertrophic *black form of behaviour* on a respective chakra, being unable to «eat» so much.

Just from apparent signs it's hard to say, how chakra got excited. For this we must analyse person's behaviour and his state during certain time. If his chakra stably stays for a long time in the excited state, probably he's not *burning it up*, but **eats** too much, i.e. takes more energy from others than he can «digest». How, for example, we can «overfeed» our Ajna? By destroying someone's worldview and giving nothing in return, making people doubt in their creeds. Having a well-developed mental apparatus it's easy to persuade anyone that he's wrong, even if it is not so. If person's worldview starts collapsing, the liberated energy comes to your «taking» Ajna, but, if its natural capacity and strength isn't enough, Ajna gets «overfed» and overexcited. With the overexcited Ajna your head feels heavy and «full» — it becomes hard to think, nothing comes to mind.

It can be very useful, if you know, how to foresee human's behaviour. For example, if someone is regularly «overeating», he'll probably overeat your energy too. In the same way of you see a person with an overexcited Manipura, it means, that he made too many people depending on him. Many people owe him, «vibrating» — pay or not to pay — they can do neither of that. Or maybe such a person with an overexcited Manipura is bearing too many people on his energy — he opened his own company, where everyone is afraid to say a word, constantly nourishing him with their Manipura, which he already can't eat. In this case you can clearly foresee that he'll try to use with you the same pattern, trying to «organise» you, make you a debtor, dependant on him.

Most of people have a stereotypic behaviour. Usually a person has a limited number of stereotypes, using it with all people around.

Let's take a brief look at the connection between chakra's state and typical diseases.

Ajna

Anatomically Ajna relates to our cerebrum, eyes, frontal and maxillary sinuses, nose and upper teeth. As other chakras Ajna can be depressed, excited, blocked and loose.

Ajna gets depressed, when a person is too often obsessed with ideas, wasting his energy. In fact obsession is wasting the energy of attention. For example, you get obsessed about what's happening at home. Your energy of attention is paid to your home, i.e. your Ajna is partly out of you. If a person has a tendency to get obsessed by many things at the same time, firstly his Ajna gets overexcited and then, after the energy is overspent, becomes constantly depressed. It can provoke dull headaches. Note that headaches can be of different kinds: pressing, pulsing, acute, dull etc. They are caused by different reasons. Migraines are caused by an overexcitement of Ajna, but even often by Svadhisthana's energy flowing to Ajna.

A dull headache and all possible aberrations, states of discoordination, the state, when a person sits down and «passes away» (he isn't lost in thoughts, because when we're thinking, our eyes are active, while in this case his eyes are empty) — all these states have to do with Ajna's depression or a big «hole» in Ajna. Such «holes» and tails can be formed when a person has made too many people dependant on his logic and worldview. For example, a hypnotist is doing a session of classic hypnosis by Sharko. «I will count till 10 and you'll fall asleep» — is a definitely Ajna's emanation, after which a person gets a suggestion. What is a «suggestion»? A hypnotist takes a part of his Ajna and «cuts it in» the Ajna of another person. Maybe someone will feel better, but a hypnotist will have less energy. Nature can't be fooled.

Very often teachers have such problems, if they teach children mostly by Ajna's suggestion: «You must do like this. You got it? Like this!!!», if teacher's Ajna isn't black or he's breaking black laws, tails in Ajna can appear and eventually charka becomes depressed, causing all the above said diseases.

Specific syndromes on Ajna — less common, but also happening, is a state of discontent, manifested by Ajna. Discontent can be expressed in different ways: by Anahata (offence), Vishuddha (grumbling, criticism). It can also be expressed by Ajna — when a person looks at the world frowningly: «Wish, I couldn't see you». Usually such state «beats» the maxillary sinuses, causing arthritis, sinusitis and caries, looseness and falling of the upper teeth. Sometimes a person can have healthy lower teeth and bad upper teeth. It is usually explained by a discontented «top» and a normal Manipura, because lower teeth are more related to Manipura, while upper teeth — with maxillary sinuses, nose and Ajna. Sometimes sportsmen's upper teeth start worsening after traumas of the nose.

There are other specific syndromes, related to Ajna. For example, the syndrome of «undercrying». A person, mostly in childhood was convicted that it's bad to cry and you should hide your feelings. Emotional energies are produced, but don't leave the body, getting stuck in the muscles related to the respective chakra. In our case — in Ajna. Tears, which weren't cried out, provoke the hypertension in ocular and some facial muscles[1], which is usually seen in the constant tension in the forehead: as if the person were slightly scowling all the time. In the long run Ajna's energy is spent (because it was blocking all these emotions, though they are Anahata's ones), it breaks Ajna down. Then a person can have problems with the headache.

The directive «Wish I couldn't see you» can be suggested as an integral program. For example, parents repeat to their child: «Wish I couldn't see you», and a kid is repeating everything after them, so he gets the same habit and doesn't «see» many things. So at the energy level he destructs his own eyes together with the liver. Sometimes this breach can cause diabetes. There is such a curious relation: eyes are connected with the liver, and liver — with eyes.

Sometimes the low density in Ajna's field can be caused by the absence of one's right to have one's own worldview. The person always listens to what others say (newspapers, books, mass media), but today they say one thing, tomorrow — another... While the energy that could be used to form one's own point of view passes away... It becomes more and more difficult to think with one's own head. If the field is loose and the chakra is weak, eventually someone will surely eat this field. That's why a person with loose Ajna always finds someone to «sit» on his Ajna. Physiologically it can cause a tic in the left eye, appearing when a person got thrust an opinion, that is not his own. Though the person can stay unconscious about it. Sometimes it happens due to excessive interest to various philosophic and esoteric systems. A certain Ajna's pantophagy. A person reads, reads, listens to everything. At the same time he lets in very different energies, without crystallizing his own worldview. The truth is that all systems of other people are little bricks, by which one have to construct his own worldview. It's his karmic task on Ajna. If he doesn't do it, he's just giving his energy to all the systems and authors, so ultimately he'll have problems with Ajna.

The same reason can explain other diseases of the head and the symptoms, located on the left side.

Actually for Ajna it's very important, if the illness is located on the right or on the left side.

---

[1] To understand, which ones, look at the mirror and see, which muscles get involved when you cry.

Vishuddha

Vishuddha is related to the thyroid and parathyroid glands, ears and everything located in the larynx, to the gullet, trachea, upper bronchus. Sometimes the problems on Vishuddha can injure upper area of the lungs (although mostly they are on Anahata), the tongue (with which we speak) and the neck-bones.

The most common state of excitement is due to the fact that a person didn't say all, he wanted. Time after time we want to say something — sometimes something pleasant, sometimes unpleasant, we have our own opinion. One's opinion must be expressed, but a person has a program, blocking his right to freely express his opinion. Nevertheless, the energy stays there, not expressed, it accumulates in Vishuddha. This causes the feeling of «a bur in the throat» — the first signal, still on the energy plane, that chakra is in trouble. Eventually this «bur» can lead to various diseases. If it's a «bur» of offence, it can cause illnesses like asthma. Bronchitis also has to do with the unsaid discontent or just with cultivating in oneself the state of resentment, but then we're speaking about Anahata states.

Sometimes Vishuddha can get excited because a person behaves himself blackly by Vishuddha, while his chakra is white. So he provokes people to get interested in some information, they get obsessed with this, the energy is coming to his Vishuddha, which can't «digest» it. As a result chakra gets excited, and the person gets diseases, caused by the hyperfunction of the respective organs.

From the point of view of logic, if chakra is excited, organs must get excited too and vice versa, but in reality it's all the other way round. **If a person gets an excited Vishuddha, he'll have a syndrome of thyroid insufficiency. And when chakra's depressed — a syndrome of overfunction.** A «goiter»[1] is a syndrome of depressed Vishuddha, not of the excited one.

A depressed Vishuddha causes asthmas, bronchitis and so on. Curiously very often Vishuddha gets depressed because of the criticism. Criticism actually has to do with some insufficiency in Manipura, but criticising, we throw out the energy of Vishuddha. Criticism is a hyperexpression of one's opinion. A person is expressing his opinion — no one asks him, but he goes on and on. It causes various kinds of a sore throat, tonsillitis, i.e. inflammatory processes in the throat. The most common reason for a sore throat is criticism: one have criticised someone, judged him, and you get a sore throat. Rinsed with eucalyptus and sea salt, it seems to get better, but in fact you should immediately find

---

[1] Hypothyroid goiter / hypothyroidism /, under which thyroid gland may be enlarged up to the rate at which the body tries to make up to its hormone functions. There is euthyroid, hyperthyroidic, goiter. Their nature is different.

out, who judged by you and where was. Criticism causes many acute disorders with teeth. After having criticised someone teeth start aching with exactly an acute pain. Periodontosis is a more complicated disease, caused by problems in different chakras.

A disease coming from Vishuddha is deafness — not inborn, but the acquired, karmic one. The reason is that the person refuses to listen to other people's opinion. You tell him something, and he just doesn't listen. This way he shuts off, closing the inflow to his chakra.

Another disorder, related to Vishuddha is stammering. By my observations stammering has to do with the breach in Vishuddha or with the fact, that Vishuddha's flow is devoured by someone else. Sometimes a kid can't pronounce all letters. In this case we have to see, who «is sitting» on his chakra (taking the energy, assigned for his development; see «Forming of chakras in childhood»). Very often isolation of the «devourer» from the child results in improvement.

The syndrome of the breached or delegated Vishuddha on the psychoemotional level is losing the aesthetic sense. A person is indifferent for how he's dressed: nicely or not, aesthetically or not, losing the interest to his own look.

Anahata

Anahata is related to the cardio-vascular system, first of all the heart itself, lungs, all thoracic vertebrae, arms and hands, ribs and all intercostal spaces, lower part of bronchus (they partly relate to Vishuddha and partly to Anahata, depending on where bronchitis is located).

The state of Anahata is easy to define, even if you don't see energies. Just take a look at the person's hand; if his palm is dry in many petty wrinkles, it usually means he has a depressed Anahata. And vice versa, if the hand is «fleshy and juicy» his Anahata is OK.

Clogged Anahata is typical for a person with the rigid sphere of feelings. A person with a clogged Anahata has no right to freely express his feelings. He can't freely love, freely hate, freely rejoice, freely grieve and so on. His feelings are «gripped in a vice» and blocked. Such a person can be easily noticed by some apparent signs, even if he has no diseases. First of all, when he is breathing the FYB or any breath at all, he doesn't breathe with his chest — only with his belly and his clavicles, his thorax being unable to widen. Secondly, there is so-called «armour» — he walks as if he were in a shell, like a monolith. Almost always it's accompanied with various symptoms of osteochondrosis, scoliosis. In fact, everywhere there is a rigidity of the back, we can usually speak about a clogged chakra. Eventually a clogged Anahata can cause heart diseases.

Further more, if a person has a blocked right to express his feelings, it results in hypertension and depression of Anahata. There are some possible ways for the disease to develop. On the one hand the depression can be caused by the fact that an unused organ atrophies. There is a general principle, the law of Lemark. On the other hand such a person can often become an object of obsession for others: «He's such an emotional retard!» This causes grudges against his Anahata, energy outflows etc. While Anahata's depression causes high blood pressure, hypertension. In perspective there is a certain possibility to end up with a heart attack. Although heart attack is a special illness. According to my observations it develops, when there are a lot of people, who got obsessed about someone at the same time, and this obsession is specific: like «Smooth sailing to the leaking boat!» When many people want to get rid of someone, annoying them. There can be other reasons. Recall the movie «Time to wish». The protagonist has a heart attack. The reason: he was living not by his own wishes, but by those of others, giving away his Anahata.

Excited Anahata can be caused by the fact, that a person attracts other people's feelings. For example, a common picture: an aged family couple, where a husband has hypertension and his wife — a hypotonia. Both have an ill heart. Complaints: «he doesn't love me anymore, doesn't understand me, doesn't care enough», and from his side: «I am so exhausted!» He feels guilty. This feeling is already a breach in Anahata. He is trying to give her as much as he can, having less and less of energy, that causes a «hole», while she doesn't really need this energy. The wife has it too much, she can't eat it, her Anahata gets excited, the blood pressure falls, the head aches.

Possible lung illnesses like pneumonia, tuberculosis etc. are caused by the lack of *joie de vivre.* It's not a coincidence that tuberculosis was a «favourite» disease of Russian aristocracy, which was brought up in sorrow: «an English spleen or Russian sorrow».

Lung illnesses are directly related to such feeling as anguish. Anguish is the lacking of Fire in lungs. Not a pure fire, but the energy of joy, vivacity. If a person can rejoice his life, it's OK. Remember the famous movie «The formula of love»? «Daddy says it's unworthy to enjoy only happiness from life». Here he was meaning a delight; Svadhisthana is a pleasure, but delight, oriented on some object, is more on Anahata. Not to forget that this Daddy was lying paralysed, which could make us doubt about his life position.

Sometimes pneumonia can happen after you seriously quarrel with someone. Swearing, saying out all the complaints can breach Anahata (with dirty energies), which in its turn can lead to lung diseases. Bronchitis happen when a person is discontented with his life. Everything seems wrong, and a person just sits and cultivates this state. If this state's local, he gets an acute bronchitis, if constant and continuous — a chronic one.

192

There can also be all possible disorders of the spine in Anahata zone: osteochondrosis, scoliosis etc. Osteochondrosis as the most «popular» disease of our time (for all my life I»ve seen not more than five people, who didn't have it), is caused by blocking or depression of the respective chakra. If it's clogged or depressed, a person stoops in the respective zone. It becomes chronic, muscles get a little inflammation, come along with the position of the spine, while the spine repeats the position of muscles. If a person has the pain, starting in his shoulders down the solar plexus, he can for sure train more liberate expression of his feelings.

Scoliosis, spinal curvatures are caused by another aspect. As it was said before, our right side is «masculine» and the left one — «feminine». When a person gets less energy on the either side, he starts stooping respectively. In this case he breaches the law like this: either he can express his feelings, but can't receive it or vice versa; or he has some definite complaints only from men or only from women, especially in the childhood, when there is a big dependence on one of one of the parents — I love my Mom very much, and I don't love my Dad — or vice versa.

The spine is arching, when chakra's excited. A person gets more energy, than he can digest.

All possible intercostal neuralgias are often related to Anahata as well, and according to my practice, they arise due to some local breaches. A person has «shoot through someone's feelings». These problems are easily treated by a manual therapy, by resetting vertebra, and in a few days the pain goes away.

Mastopathy also has to do with blocked Anahata's feelings. It can happen to women, who have a lot of feelings and can't express them. It's a stagnation of Anahata energy — inside it's boiling up, and outside there is nothing. According to my observation, sometimes it happens in overdisciplined families. For example, when a father holds his daughter in iron hands. Feelings are not blocked, when if a woman has them, she expresses it, if not — doesn't, but when she has energy and doesn't emanate it, mastopathy is quite possible.

In the young age girl can have mastopathy, because she's ready to starts her sex life, but doesn't do it. Such mastopathy if not disregarded, passes after she finds herself a regular partner. Because in our society such beliefs as «no sex before marriage», she'd better do everything in time.

In our times there are many young people with a deformed thorax, and in general upper Anahata is very rare. Anahata has several segments. Upper Anahata is responsible for love to God, Nature, Cosmos — transcendent love — *bhakti*. Middle Anahata is responsible for love, friendship with equals, for partnership. And the low Anahata is responsible for love to «one's own»: my home, my dog, my wife. A person is stooping by a zone, which is depressed. Nowadays upper Anahata is very rare, while the low Anahata sometimes comes out. That's why young people usually have a «black walk» — like that of rap singers. You can't explain how to love God to a person, who doesn't have this segment of Anahata.

On the psycho-emotional level the syndrome of breached Anahata is depression and touchiness.

Manipura

Manipura relates to such viscera: stomach, gastrointestinal tract (except for the upper gullet), intestines — in the first place the small intestine, because large is more related to Muladhara; upper area of kidneys and adrenals (with their adrenaline and so on); liver, spleen, spine at the level of Manipura; pancreas.

Depressed Manipura is formed when a person is constantly «plying» and is always «pressed» by others. Such person has no habit to take responsibility for his actions and always lays it on someone else. He is inclined to live on credit. He is unable to stand upon his interests.

Manipura is responsible for dominating, for person's capacity to dominate over others. If this capacity is weak or blocked, a person delegates his Manipura energy to someone else. What they turn him back, is what he «eats». If he's always giving more than he has, he gets constantly depressed and forms an image of a «small guy», and his Manipura consequently gets depressed too. Medicine calls this state a psychological stress. A person always feels anxiety like «how will I live?» Fears are all syndromes of the breached Manipura.

When we lose Manipura energy, we feel scared and anxious. The breached, depressed Manipura causes first of all acidity and gastritis. An ulcer is a result of accepting a foreign position, dictated from someone else. He'd like to change, but he can't, being unable to assert himself — and the ulcer is assured. In psychology there is a conception that ulcer is the autoagression. When a person is bullied, aggression arises in him, but he can't express it to the other person, so he expresses it on himself.

Liver disorders are usually caused by human's rage, expressed or not. A person cherishes his ill-will and even feels «high». Liver and gall-bladder are «husband-and-wife» in Chinese system. If person's liver gets excited, gall-bladder ducts get depressed. Bile isn't produced intensively, gets inspissated, flakes appear in the inspissated bile and stick together, forming gallstones.

194

All possible disorders in pancreas, like pancreatitis, are cause by various Manipura breaches. My personal statistics in this is little, but the most possible reason of many diseases is the absence of the inside right for the initiative. A person is good, he has Manipura, but to take the initiative, to make something on his own (low Manipura) — he can get illnesses of pancreas.

Duodenum diseases are illnesses of a depressed Manipura, autocriticism. I didn't notice any radical differences from the ordinary ulcer.

Curiously, Manipura's illness is diabetes. The reason is a general discontent with life, everything is just not right, — hence, there is no «inside burning».

Diseases of excited Manipura. A tendency to solve problems only by Manipura, a state of «eternal warrior». It can be caused by a clogged Anahata or Svadhisthana. Such people typically have a red face and dryish constitution. With Anahata and/or Svadhisthana the capillary network gets overexcited and capillaries start breaking. Manipura gets excited, and in this case acidity lowers. A person emanates too much of Manipura energy, keeping nothing inside. Such person gets a hypersensitive stomach and has the tendency to «eat something bad».

Another interesting moment: the incapacity to conceive is often explained by a depressed Manipura. If a patient has a breached Manipura (especially with her father), she can have problems in conceiving. Although a womb is located in Svadhisthana, it's connected with the fetus through Manipura, so apparently energy goes to a fetus through mother's Manipura, not Svadhisthana. If Manipura is depressed the fetus can't get energy from the start, a woman gets pregnant, but has miscarriages. She needs to get off her Manipura whoever is sitting on it, to become independent from other people's opinions, conceptions, relations, to feel independent and free. From the karmic point of view it's obvious; if a person isn't independent and free, a newborn baby will become psychologically defective. Who needs it? So the soul, wanting to reincarnate, ignores such parents.

Svadhisthana

With Svadhisthana are related genitals (male and female), bladder, lower part of kidneys, renal pelvises, ureters, urethra, ovaries, womb for women, lower back (except for the coccyx, related to Muladhara), hips.

The most common mistake is to promise, «loosening» Svadhisthana fields and their non-realisation. A man or a woman have «spread» their fields, others got obsessed, prepared themselves for sex, and get nothing. The essence of this mistake is blocking one's desire, forbidding oneself to derive pleasure. Want to do it — do it, but, if a person has a desire, but gives oneself no right to have it, sooner or later he'll have problems with health. Women have ill appendages, inflammation in ovaries.

The next mistake is interesting. European society is based on Christianity, so our culture has a general directive for a negative attitude towards sex. This directive lies so deep in our culture, that sometimes you can think that everything's alright and permitted, but it rests inside, staying very deep in our mentality and is very difficult to stub up. If this directive shows up actively, a person can have various mycoses (thrush and so on). On the other hand, if the person can't just groove, get his pleasure, live his thrills to the full, he can have various congested diseases, for men for example, prostatitis. Besides, due to inner limitations, one can have pain in the lower back and bad flexibility in this zone.

Another psychological reason causing different Svadhisthana diseases, is the fear to become pregnant, and for men — the fear for their woman. This can cause different illnesses, inflammations.

Syndromes of the excited Svadhisthana. Svadhisthana can become excited when a person has a lot of energy on it, but it doesn't go out by «tails» and isn't realized. A person has a desire, but «don't spread his tails». This can cause cystitis — the inflammation of the bladder. It can be the reason of blood rush to the head, of headaches, migraines, so it's the syndrome of excited Svadhisthana, when a person can't let his energy out of Svadhisthana.

This is also the reason for many schizophrenias, formed in pubertal age, when a girl is ready to start her sex life, but her family gags her with «you can't do it, it's too early». There is such disorder as flush. A girl is sitting, and suddenly her face becomes red as tomato. The reason is the same. It all passes, if she finds a regular partner, who satisfies her.

Possible desires, that appeared and weren't realized, can accumulate in hips in the form of hip contractions. Men usually get it in the anterior part of the hips, and women — in the posterior part, causing cellulite. Women have the syndrome of obesity because of the non-realized Svadhisthana.

Disorders of prostate gland are caused by the absence of the inner right to derive pleasure, by emotional rigidity — not sensational rigidity, but the emotional one. A man can't fully enjoy a woman, let himself go in sex, so he is constantly looking for new partners: tried one — it's not good, looks for another, again something doesn't work. While the problem lies inside — he has no right for a complete pleasure. Sometimes this contraction is motivated by a wish to «show himself» in the bed, to prove his men potency. The result is the same — prostatitis.

196

Fibromas, cysts and similar diseases are caused by the fact, that some men get obsessed about a woman, sometimes there is a delusion, which can be of two types — of oneself and of a man. In one case a man gets obsessed, in another — a woman pretends that she is alright.

Muladhara

We have already naturally come to it, because infertility problems have to do with Muladhara, not with Svadhisthana. Muladhara relates to the coccyx, prostate gland, pelvis, large intestines, rectum. The typical disease from Muladhara is haemorrhoids. Usually it's caused by greediness. **Greediness is overemanating one's energy on things.** What is emanating of Muladhara? A person lets his energy field out and believes, that a thing belongs to him. He spreads his field and is holding all things by it. I have one friend who suffers from haemorrhoids. He says that as soon as he gets a new attack of haemorrhoids, he throws something away, and immediately feels better. Greediness causes various problems with intestines, sometimes to constipations.

And vice versa, not holding the function of Muladhara, problems with this chakra can cause diarrhoea, although usually the reason is in Manipura. It's the incapacity of Manipura to «digest» energies. Muladhara is responsible for material things, the element of Earth. To Muladhara relate problems of bad teeth, fragile bones, sometimes arthritis, arthrosis etc. Arthritis, arthrosis is a joint tissue involvement, caused by such a purely Muladhara feature as stubbornness — a person can't give in his principles.

Muladhara is responsible for trombophlebitis and other diseases of dense blood, which is an excess of Earth in the body. Muladhara is responsible for hypersensitivity. It can be the opposite — you point at someone, and he's feeling, where exactly you pointed. This is Muladhara's weakness. The element of Earth stabilises physical, etheric and astral bodies. Earth element is present on the physical, etheric and astral planes.

I had patients — yogins, who were practicing for a long time and frustrated themselves Muladharas. Muladhara needs material possessions, safety. «My home is my fortress» is the image of Muladhara person. Instead they said «We are yogins, we don't need anything, the material world is not for us» and threw away everything from their homes, stopped taking care of their lives. In other words, a person has completely refused all Muladhara emanations. First they got a syndrome of hypersensitivity, and then started losing their teeth.

NOTE. That I always say about reasons causing illnesses, as about possible ones. With every person you must look for his particular reasons.

Rehabilitation of field's integrity and chakra stabilisation

Therapeutic complexes of asanas

Basing on the chakra conception of diseases described above, we can understand the principle of building a therapeutic complex. Such complex has for a goal «smoothing» of the field, energizing depressed chakras and sadation (removing the excess of energy) of the excited ones. If a chakra is excited because of its rigidity and the accumulated non-realized energy, one have also to work with the situation on the astral plane, i.e. to use astral techniques in asanas — to moan, to re-act one's pain and so on. The next step is to cleanse channels in the etheric plane. The criteria of successful practice are various sensations: pricking, a feeling like numbness, vibration, feeling of the energy, liberating from the respective zone. After that you can start working directly with chakras.

Note that, if chakra is depressed, at the respective level of the etheric plane there will be a «hole» ahead and a «bump» on the back. This means, you need exercises that work with both of them. The general principle of pumping the hole to a bump is the same that we used in common complexes: **the energy moves from the strained zone to the stretched one.** In order to change a hole into a bump you need some stretchings in the zone of the hole and some muscle strains in the zone of the bump.

If a chakra is depressed, to stimulate it, i.e. to fill it from the front, you should do some anterior-stretching exercises for this chakra. It can be Bhujangasana or Ushtrasana with an accent on the needed chakra.

If your chakra is excited, you have a «hole» on the back and a «bump» ahead, so you have to do some bending exercises, «squeezing» the excited etheric zone.

As it was already said in the chapter about strengthening poses, overworked chakra becomes loose, i.e. it easily loses energy. Especially, if a person didn't work on his behavioural reasons of the illness, didn't take off his «tails». In order to make energy stay in the, pumped «hole» — no matter, in the front or back part of the body, — it should be fixed by strengthening asanas for this zone.

The effect from asanas is fixed by rhythmic breathing and by other pranayamas. In the case of depressed chakras pranayamas should

198

be done before the therapeutic complex to attract additional energy to the body. It's good to do such toning pranayamas as Bhastrikas. Ideally, breathing you involve muscles of the problem zone. If you work with the excited chakra, it makes sense to do a full yoga breath in the relaxed state after a complex.

Thus **a minimum therapeutic complex, aiming stabilisation of chakra, contains three exercises: stretching, firming and pranayama.** This set should be repeated several times in the row at one pace.

The effect from this set can be slightly increased, if you add a pivoted pose accenting on the zone, you are working with. Pivoting poses enhance the energy flow, that's why they can be useful for both depressed and excited chakras.

In general all possible illnesses, caused by osteochondrosis, in the neck, thorax or lower back (radiculitis), mostly are cured by Arthamatsiendrasana and other pivoted poses (on conditions that the spine keeps the right posture).

> **WARNING!** The contrary is also true. Arthamatsiendrasana with the stooping back causes osteochondrosis. And that is very quickly. It's explained by traumatising of intervertebral disks by the simultaneous pivoting and pressing (physically), and by energy stuck in the stooping area (energy level). In less serious cases, with the chakra rigid or loose, but yet neither depressed nor excited, less exercises can be enough. In this case the minimum complex is as follows. For a loose chakra: a strengthening pose and an intensive pranayama (Bhastrika) — to calm down the excessive tension (if you succeeded in achieving it). For a rigid chakra — a stretching pose with the deep (with Muladhara set-up) rhythmical breathing with emotional reacting (moaning) and a smooth breathing to redistribute the energy, liberated from the block.

Chakras stabilisation by breathing

Chakra's depression or excitation influence on how intensively we inhale and exhale by the respective zone. Thus, **if a chakra is depressed, the person has a tendency to make a deeper exhalation** — as if he were getting rid of the air. The example of it can be someone, sighing with his chest, when he has a breached Anahata (i.e. being in depression). This point of view is proved by the opinion of Anatoliy Petrovich Zilber, professor, MD: «...the most of «breathing chronics» especially with prevailing obstructive[1] disorders (hampering the air pass — *comment of Safronov*) have a breathing pattern with an active inhalation, whereas it needs to be passivated».

---

[1]   Such diseases, like bronchial asthma, are usually caused by chakra's depression.

On the contrary **a person with the excited chakra has a tendency to a deeper inhalation**, as if he didn't want to let the air go.

The contrary is also true: chakra can be stabilised by changing the habitual breathing pattern, i.e. by activising the inhalation and passivating the exhalation for a depressed chakra and passivating inhalation and making more active the exhalation for an excited one. Of course, the most significant effect will be achieved, if you work with breathing muscles at the level of the problem chakra.

The easiest way to use this method is by practicing rhythmic breathing, but it can also be done with any pranayama, including intensive ones.

Affecting meridian system by yoga exercises

How it was already said, asanas influence not only on our viscera, but also on the system of musculotendinous meridians (see Appendix 1). The localisation of meridians is so that they often come quite far from zones, on which they influence. That's why many asanas make an indirect impact on organs, physically not involved in them. For example, sarpasana stretches the stomach meridian, padahastasana — the one of the bladder, all pivoted poses — meridians of gall-bladder.

Like chakras, every meridian can be in an «excessive» (excited) and «insufficient» (depressed) state[1]. In the first case the pain symptom appears when you squeeze the meridian, in the second — when you stretch it.

Stretching meridians, we stimulate them. Basing on this fact and knowing main principles of acupuncture, you can make complexes for a precise treating of chosen organs.

---

[1] For more details about excessive and insufficient aspects of meridians and organs see a classic monograph of Tabeeva D. M. «Manual of reflex acupuncture». Of course this theory is a view of Chinese classic doctors of the balance of ANS branches, while tables given by Tabeeva is a detailed and more ancient variation of Wein tables.

Harmonisation of ANS balance by asymmetric types of breathing and asanas

Almost all basic asanas and pranayamas equally influence on Ida and Pingala, are symmetric in their kind and presume that a practitioner is also symmetric, though most of people are not (remember your last visit to photographer: «Sit straighter, you shoulder up, your chin up...»).

The disbalance of ANS branches is also seen in body's asymmetry. Because sympathetic and parasympathetic ANS branches are related to Ida and Pingala, which are projected on the right and left nostril, their disbalance at the level of any chakra results in the fact, that people unconsciously take asymmetric poses, thinking that they sit still and straight.

The main principle of how subtle bodies project on the physical is that a person are usually closing the zone, which is breached and lacks energy. It concerns not only bending ahead (stooping in the respective zone), but also all possible unconscious lateral bendings. For example, if a person lacks for energy in the left channel at the level of Vishuddha, he'll be always looking a little bit to the left, and the same with the right side; lacking for energy in one of the channels in Anahata, he'll slightly drop one shoulder; in Svadhisthana — he'll throw ahead one hip etc.

The uneven distribution of energy can be seen by asymmetry of the feet. There is a law of «accumulation of mistakes»: the further from the source, the better you see all initial mistakes. Ida and Pingala go from the top down, so the more down, the more obvious is the asymmetry. It explains, for example, why some people can easily sit in one-sided half-lotus, and can't change the leg for another side.

The most common problem is an unconscious turning of the head, which has to do with the excessive «kha» (right) and «tkha» (left) petal of Ajna. Once more, **a person himself thinks he's sitting still and straight**.

The contrary is also true: this or another ANS branch can be activated by changing the symmetry of the pose and by changing the balance of breathing intensity by different nostrils. For examples, sympatics can be recommended to do breathing exercises not in a common position, but turning their head slightly to the right, i.e. activating the left channel. They can also make longer stays in right-sided poses (where the head is turned to the right), like sarpasana, Arthamatsiendrasana etc.

201

Pivoting our body at the level of a chakra, we can influence quite precisely on our body. Doing asymmetric pranayamas, like Akapalabhati, you can breathe with just one nostril.

Some Indian sources recommend activating the needed type of breathing by putting a cotton tampon in one nostril, doing exercises, but I personally think, this method is too extreme and can be hardly recommended as therapeutic.

The asymmetry principle can also be used in doing asanas. For example, if a person has an active left channel, he can be advised to do yoga-mudra not straight, but with a slight (10–15°) turning of the body on the left side. Although even a conscious straightening in asanas, distorted by the pathologic asymmetry of the channels, already gives a certain harmonising effect.

Awareness is the main clue to yoga and it's even more true for yoga-therapy.

YOGA
AND NUTRITION

Probably there is no other subject that would be so intricate and contradictory, as the healthy nutrition. On the one hand (and it can be proved by one's own experience), nutrition influences greatly on our physical and emotional state. On the other, it would take many pages just to enumerate all existing «healthy diets». The saddest thing is that most of them are contradictory. Moreover I know many cases, when a diet which was good for one person, bringing him health and strength, turned out to be very harmful for another. Apparently, people are indeed different and should eat differently. So a single universal system of nutrition for everyone doesn't exist. However there are some principles, basing on which one can build his own diet.

Principles of nutrition of all bodies

As it was already said, yoga distinguished eight human bodies, four of them being «mortal», collapsing after human's death, have to be fed.

Physical body lives on fats, proteins, carbohydrates, microelements, vitamins and on other substances, which must be well-balanced.

Etheric body lives on the etheric energy, in particular, from food. To be rich in etheric energy, food must be «alive», i.e. as natural as possible, being as less processed and stored as possible. For example, greens, grown in one's own garden without chemicals, are more alive, than «hydroponics» ones. Fresh meat is more alive, that the one that's been frozen, and even more than the canned one (absolutely dead product). The degree of «life» in a product can be defined by seeing the size and quality of its etheric — alive products usually have it bigger and denser. There is an easier way to see it. Alive products go bad slower, than the same dead ones (if they weren't specially processed — in which case they can't be taken at all). For example, greens, picked from one's own garden can stay fresh for 2-3 days, while «hydroponics» look faded by the same night — because they don't have much etheric.

If etheric body is underfed, it gets exhausted, its vitality falls, and the person becomes sickly. In my opinion, such problems of the modern civilisation as the chronic fatigue syndrome, allergy — are all results of underfeeding etheric body.

Astral body is nourished by impressions, i.e. by tastes. Once dieticians made a test: feeding a person by a well balanced, but one-taste food. So the volunteer became ill, because his astral body wasn't nourished. That is why mankind throughout its history was paying so much attention to the taste of the food. That's why the restaurant food, filled with astral bodies of the personnel, specifically decorated, costs more, than the home one (although the home one tastes better).

There is food with just an astral component and no physical and etheric one, like for example, spices, flavour additives, beverages like «Coca-Cola», derived chemically.

Understanding principles of nutrition of the bodies explains one of the roots of another serious problem of nowadays — the obesity. An average city dweller has no bright and various impressions, so he is emotionally hungry. One of the ways to satisfy this hunger is food, but it turns out that food has not only astral, but also a physical component... From this we can conclude that one of the ways to fight obesity is to fill one's life with good and diverse impressions. Better not «canned» (from TV).

Mental body lives on thoughts and ideas. «Knowledge is food» says «Siva sutra». That's why humanity continuously creates new dishes (as if the old ones weren't enough), and the most expensive one in the restaurant is «the chef's special». These dishes contain mental energy, the energy of creativity. Nevertheless mental body nourishes mostly not by food, but with ideas and information.

The principle of food's correspondence to the constitutional type

As it was already said, different people should eat differently. Already the laws of Manu, representatives of different casts were advised to have different diets and restrictions in eating. One of the systems, helping to choose one's own diet is the Ayurvedic system of three doshas.

Dosha — is one of the basic principles of Indo-Tibetan medicine. *Vata, pita, kapha* — Wind, Bile and Phlegm — are three basics of the human body. The balance of these doshas determines the constitutional type of a person. Knowing one's type you can adjust your way of life, your diet, individual practice, in order to achieve a perfect balance. Indo-Tibetan medicine believes that vata appeared due to the merging of Wing (vayiu) and the Ether (akasha), pita — from Fire (agni) and Water (apo), kapha — from Water (apo) and Earth (pritkhvi). The prevalence of dosha, up to the percent ratio, can be determined by person's constitutional type. Ayurveda has specific diet recommendations for every prevailing dosha.

The principle of using gunas

It's well known, that Indian tradition was using three basic states (gunas), in which every system, including a man, can be. These states are called *sattva, rajas* and *tamas*.

Sattvic are fresh fruit, vegetables, greens, couched grain, fresh natural dairy products, natural (not chemical) sweets.

Rajas are spices and flavours, spicy food, fresh steamed meat, some types of alcohol (high quality cognac, tequila).

Tamastic are all canned products, roots (like potato), meat, fat, alcohol like beer etc.

Eating products from either group puts you in a state, corresponding to a guna. Some Indian texts, especially religious ones, recommend only sattvic food, but there can be life situations, where not sattva should be prevailing. For example, active efforts need a lot of rajas. Sometimes after too intensive spiritual practices and physical activity one needs to «get back to Earth», and this can be done by tamas.

You should also remember, that person's belonging to a certain *varna* also determines his best diet. Thus the prevailing guna in brahmin's nutrition (meaning that he has an occupation, corresponding his caste), should be sattva, for kshatriya — rajas, for vaishya — rajas and tamas and for shudra — tamas.

The structure of nutrition also differs by castes. Hence, brahmin should eat a little, but various food, while shudra should eat a lot.

The principle of time and place

Our body is a result of many millions of evolution. In this evolution we adapted ourselves to eat according to seasons of the natural Sun cycle. Hundred years ago refrigerators were invented along with other advanced methods of storage, and for the first time the diet has become independent from the season, but our body is still used to it. That's why it's better to take for a basis of your nutrition products, that nature of your region is giving at the present season. If it's spring, you should eat greens, if it's summer — berries, vegetables, fruit, autumn — grains and roots, winter — meat dishes. It's also important, because «alive» products that you eat are directly connected to their «relatives». I remember once we had such a big crop of apples, that we managed to keep it till the late spring, but the day, when apple-trees started blossoming, all the rest of the old-year crop has rotted — once and completely. Which proved one more time, that the food we eat contains its own information and lives its life. We shouldn't neglect it.

So **the optimum food is supposed to be the one, grown in your region**[1]. Nature is an interrelated homeostatic system, providing its children with all they need, the way they need. That's why the food, grown in your land contains energies and substances you need for life. Of course, I don't propose to forget about bananas and oranges, but we shouldn't neglect this principle.

---

[1]   An indirect proof of this principle is the following medical fact: Europeans have most food allergies to citruses and chocolate, i.e. from products, grown on other continents, while Africans are never allergic to citruses.

206

The principle of following one's natural wishes

No doubt, human's body is a complicated self-organising system, which probably should know itself, which products it needs, and which ones are bad. In early childhood it is really so. In a famous experiment a little kid was given a lot of different food (put in the room, where he was closed). He was crawling and tasting everything. When researches counted what was eaten, it turned out to be perfectly balanced, although from adult's point of view taste combinations were awful. Where does this capacity go, when we grow old? **It is destructed by the imposed stereotypes of nutrition**[1]. That's why, if a person, being more than 5 years old, for the worse burdened with diseases, decides to eat what he wants, he just makes his problems worse. You can come back to natural nutrition only after having seriously cleansed your body. Your physical body — from slags, your psyche — from food habits, from beliefs about what one «should eat». Lately it also became crucial to cleanse our astral body from all desires, induced by advertisement — «to eat something» or «to try something».

One of the best ways to cleanse our body and psyche is fasting. After the correct coming from fasting our body temporary gets back the capacity to see, which food is healthy for it. Very often after fasting products that used to be desirable for us (like complex pastry) become disgusting even by their look, but after a while our body gets dirty again and starts demanding more and more pervert food.

By the way, these criteria can be taken as the instrument to see, whether it's not time to fast. If you want to eat «something, you don't even know, what», your body urgently needs fasting.

In addition to fasting yoga proposes many so-called «cleansings» of the body, which we'll not discuss here, because they are perfectly described in Ar Eddar's (Vasiliev's) book «The treatise on nutrition». Here are just some principles of health-improving fasting.

---

[1] For example, before 6 month age, we have no salt receptors, but, if you start putting salt in your food, they form very quickly. Besides parents are often busy, so they give their kids canned baby food instead of healthy natural one. Due to all this children develop food allergy — first monocomponent, then multicomponent. With time it progresses into neurodermatitis, pollinosis and bronchial asthmas. Curiously, if parents follow doctor's instructions and don't give their child the allergen product for 6–12 months, very often the body «forgets» about this allergen and later on shows no reaction on it.

Principles of health-improving fasting

1. Fasting is better done during a full moon or on a new moon.

2. Don't overeat the day before fasting. Better don't eat meat. In the evening dine with kefir and give yourself an enema.

3. During fasting it is **forbidden to:**

    — brush teeth (especially, if fasting is long);

    — take medications;

    — smoke, drink alcohol etc.

    — overwork.

4. During fasting it is **obligatory to:**

    — drink water (2-3 litres a day);

    — give enema every evening;

    — cleanse your tongue and mouth;

    — stay in the open air.

5. During fasting it's **recommended to:**

    — practice yoga (better in first half of the day);

    — if you freeze, take a hot bath (if your heart is strong) or a shower;

    — if your head aches, give an additional enema or cleanse your stomach (provoke vomiting).

6. **Recovering from fasting should last as much as the fasting itself.** The wrong recovering ruins the positive effect from fasting. It is done in three steps, approximately equal in time:

    — drinking diluted juice (gradually replacing water with juice). **Don't drink** orange fruit and carrots juice;

    — eating vegetable salads (without dressing);

    — eating cooked cereals (no salt or butter).

After fasting it is not recommended to eat meat and non-dietary products for the time that equals the time of fasting.

YOGA AND SEX. SEX PRACTICIES IN YOGA

«This world is born in passion and with passion it liberates».

Hevadjra Tantra

The subject of this chapter is obviously very complicated and deserves a whole book, that's why we'll just make some general notes, or better say warnings, that can help the practitioners avoid some biggest troubles.

Modern «about-yoga» circles have two opposite attitudes to sex. Some (especially Indian) sources have a very negative attitude to sex, propagating *brahmacharia* — a complete or partial continence (out of marriage or for than conceiving a baby). This belief was formed under the influence of religious doctrines, from the so to say «religionising» of yoga, quite significantly distorting its genuine spirit. All contemporary religions somehow demonise sex, because, clogging people's Svadhisthana, religious egregors live on this non-realised energy. Ancient religious were less dramatic about sex, though they also were using sexual energy for their, mostly magical, goals. All peoples had their festivals of fertility, accompanied with group orgies, vivid sexual demonstrations, tabooed in everyday life. Remember Thais from Athens, who gave herself on the ploughed field to increase fecundity. Ancient Slavs also had such rituals, they were using the Svadhisthana energy, received by sexual games and the group sex to call the rain in the agricultural period (Ivana Cupala).

Studying ancient Indian sources, like Mahabharata or even older «The ocean of the streams of stories» by Somadeva (approximately the V century B.C.), we can see, that they don't have that typical Indian Puritanism. Yogins and ascetics in these stories are living in ashrams with their wives, falling in love with apsaras and simply beautiful women and so on. Gods of the Indian pantheon behave the same way. In the ancient Indian culture sex isn't made a fetish, neither demonised. It's treated as something natural, though its power is known and used. In particular, with magical goals:

209

«A woman is indeed a Fire, her Womb is her fuel. The hair is its smoke. Her genitals — the flame. Coming inside — carbons. Pleasure — sparkles. On this fire gods make a sacrifice of a semen».

Brihadaraniaka Upanishada

It's also interesting, that the term *brahmacharia* is almost always interpreted as «continence», while it's really translated as «apprenticeship by brahmin» (*acharia* in Sanskrit means apprentice) and doesn't directly relate to the continence.

So where did Indian schools get their unhealthy Puritanism? It seems, that this question has several answers. First of all it was the influence of Islam and later Christianity in times when India was conquered. Secondly it's a result of perception of the Western people, seeing Indian ideas through their own prism. And finally, the objective problem of deesoterisation of yoga, free access for everyone to previously closed schools, forcing to hide the most efficient techniques of work, replacing them (to avoid serious problems) by widely understandable «religious bubblegum».

There is another branch of «studying» sexual practices. Every more or less educated person «knows» that Tantra is the sex yoga (though it's not), has read Kamasutra, which he thinks has to do with Tantras (which is also not true), thinks that in the Eastern world there were spiritual practices, using sex (though they are in all cultures, including the European one). Some people heard about «Tao of love» and Chinese techniques of sex without ejaculation. Some even practice it themselves, mistakenly taking it for Indian vadjroli mudra. In more simple versions of modern «tantra», sex is practiced for sexual liberation, which is great, but more relates to psychotherapy, than to esoterics or yoga. This is the problem of all mentioned beliefs. What neophytes think is the ancient practice, at the best is its shade and extremely simplified forms, with no true sense. Some of them can play dirty tricks. For example, pseudotaoistic practices of sex without ejaculation with raising energy, result in sex, reduced to a simple mechanic and ether-oriented procedure. «Five thousand love pushes» don't differ from ordinary jogging or any other physical routine. The emotional (astral) component of making love is lost, causing a rapid destruction of Svadhisthana and poor astral body. One just doesn't want to make love anymore... Of course, Taoists knew, how to avoid this trouble, but «forgot» to say. Still these are esoteric techniques. Another dirty trick has to do with the fact, that without compensating exercises (at least nauli), practicing sex without ejaculation causes congestions in prostate, which eventually can cause prostatitis. Another dirty trick of this technique is that is blocks the natural energy flow between a man and a woman. A man doesn't give energy, and a woman, giving her energy, soon grows old. Karmic debts are forming...

210

The same with modern «tantra». **Classic tantra** is a technique of development of the astral body. All tantra rituals (not only sexual ones) cultivate the capacity to feel, to have different emotional states in their peak forms. Tantric techniques don't include ejaculation control, they aim to get the most acute strong sensations, to know how to feel them, staying conscious. Tantra uses many instruments, sex is just one of them, all aiming to develop sensitivity. Take for example, the ritual pancha-tattva: a person breaks all taboos and ritually derives pleasure with different chakras. In India devoted brahmins don't eat meat, don't smoke stimulants, don't practice group sex and so on — these are their traditional taboos.

In the ritual they do all on the contrary: drink wine (religious Hindu never drinks wine — for him it's like drinking urine for us), then they eat meat, fish, smoke marijuana and have group sex. A person is living through some peak states due to breaking taboo, but does a modern person feel the same way, drinking and smoking in everyday basis? For him such a ritual would bring no peak sensations, and would become just a way to «party». It's a mistake to take tantra for debauch. The difference is that in tantra rituals peak states are achieved to learn how to consciously control this energy. While in debauch a person doesn't learn to consciously control energies.

The degree of control of astral energies is determined by his capacity to keep consciousness, and not only in his fantasy, but in real life, where these energies are present. For instance, you may be thinking that you keep «brahmacharia», sitting in an isolated cell, cold and damp, but when you have essential scents around together with naked women, this belief can prove to be wrong.

This concerns all chakras. A person controls his states, until his chakra contains more energy, he can deal with. That's why to develop chakra you need to work with peak states. That's what real tantra is about. Of course, you also need some practice to acquire your experience of these states, to harmonically «include» their results in your everyday life. Tantra had it, but do modern «tantrists» have it[1]?

So what is the real attitude of yoga to the problem of sex? Obviously it comes from the essence of yoga itself: **yoga is mastering of energy.** Including sexual energy, which means mastering one's desire, sensations and orgasm.

For a man this means the capacity to lift his sexual energy without ejaculation, and for a woman — to lift her energy whenever she wants it, i.e. provoke her own orgasm. The level of control of sexual energy for men is seen at how long he can make love. For a woman it's the contrary — how fast she can feel the orgasm making love. Both

---

[1]   About changed states of consciousness and the problem of their acquiring you can read in my monograph «Religious psychopracticies in the history of culture».

depend on how channels are clean and on the capacity to lift one's energy. Control of the etheric energy for man is his capacity to raise it by his anterior middle channel, and for a woman it's the capacity to keep moving, feeling the orgasm without «losing» it.

However sexual energy control isn't only about sex. Sexual energy motivates people for many actions. Becoming aware of these motives, defining them is also an element of controlling subtle energy.

If used correctly, sexual energy gives us many siddhas. By sexual energy you can attract anyone, because almost everyone reacts on it. «The one who is reflecting everyday on Svadhisthana, becomes the master of love and affection», says «Siva samhita».

Sexual energy influences the animals. If a person's Svadhisthana is at least a little bit open, he finds contact with animals. For example, a dog of the opposite sex stops barking, a person is no longer an aggressive object for it. Sexual energy influences the plants[1]. Besides, it's almost a universal healing energy, related, as it was already said, to the element of Water.

An important aspect of sexual practices including tantra is partners' exchange of energy, and not just the astral, but also with etheric one. Men and women are indeed bearers of absolutely different astral energies. A man bears in himself a spiritual-regulating energy, while a woman — the energy of activity and desire. A mutual nourishing of partners with these energies can significantly harmonise both, although unfavourable energy exchange is also possible — when the balance seriously shifts to either side. Too much of «male» energy makes sex too vapid and «rational». Physically it shows by the fact, that woman (and later her man) will fear to express her desires. Too much of «female» energies make the man «lose his head». He'll be knocked out by emotions (not always positive) and this pair will lose its spiritual core. This is also a problem for sex with numerous partners.

Sex of a man with several women is energetically interesting for all participants (and as a result emotionally pleasant), only if his «men's» pith is strong enough to control the total emotionality of all his women-partners. As for woman, practicing sex with several men, her sexual desire must be stronger than their unconscious competitiveness. If this rule is violated, there can be energy (and other) problems.

Notice that this rule applies not only to a group sex, i.e. a direct and simultaneous energy exchange between participants, but also to situations, where a person has several partners, who don't even know each other.

An important component of esoteric tantra is practicing sex in transpersonal states, helping to develop astral body.

---

[1]   To prove it you can just put a weak plant on your bed.

212

Hatha-yoga for Svadhisthana

Legs, especially their stretching relate to Svadhisthana. Usually a person with the «easy» emotional sphere can easily do splits, does padahastasana, and vice versa, if he can't do it, he has emotional blocks in Svadhisthana. Usually the opposite is also true: correct stretching helps to open Svadhisthana fields.

To «wind up» Svadhisthana's field, a good exercise is hips rotation. It can be different. When we are rotating till the limit of Muladhara set up, to feel strain in every point of rotation, after a while we are feeling the heat in the belly. Another similar exercise is when you rotate your hips, but not till the limit, instead you «send» them to rotate automatically, as if it didn't depend on you. Rotate and then let go to make your hips move mechanically. This exercise helps to use Svadhisthana independently from the third eye. People with a strong third eye find it difficult to let go their emotional sphere liberally with no control.

Another exercise is called «Tibetan pendulum». It is based on the same principle, as the second one, but hips aren't rotated. A person stands straight, clenches fists, fixes them in one point and starts doing alternate-reciprocal motion by the lower part of his body. This exercise should be done for a long time — up to half an hour, non-stop. Inertial rhythm raises the energy.

In all described exercises it's important, that the «push» goes «from the earth», not from the body. If it's not so, it means, that the person uses in sex not the natural energy, but the energy of his mind, i.e. he's motivated not by his own desire. Such sex is exhaustive.

Men can cleanse their Svadhisthana from non-realised desires by Ushtrasana. This pose also favours the capacity to make sexual intercourse longer and so on. For women it's viparita karani. Men accumulate non-realised sexual energy in the anterior part of their hips, while women — in the posterior part, in their buttocks. If a woman has painful points on her buttocks, it means, she has a non-realised sexual energy.

YOGA AND THE STARS

Generally speaking, astrology is a separate branch of esoteric knowledge, a powerful instrument (in skilful hands) of cognising oneself and the world. To study astrology one needs time and system approach, that's why in this book we'll only give some general notions about how celestial bodies influence on your hatha yoga session.

How moon cycles influence on our body

It's commonly believed that the Moon, turning around the Earth, influences on how fluidities move in our planet in general (high and low tide), as well as in biological objects. People are exposed to this power too. Thus we can notice that there is a specific movement of vital energy in the body, reminding high and low tides in nature: the excessive energy makes a whole round of the human's body during 28 days. The nature of these «high tides» is still unknown, but we can presume, that the physiology of this phenomena has to do with filling the capillaries with blood, when «the tide becomes high» in the respective zone. Indeed astrologists have noticed long time ago, that at certain phases of the Moon, certain organs become more vulnerable to different diseases. In this time it's also not recommended to do surgery on these organs because of the great risk of blood loss, the bleeding, which is difficult to stop.

Besides in the zone of «high tide» some other functions get activated, for example, the respective zone becomes more erogenic.

When the Moon is full, the most energies are concentrated in the head, and when it's new — in the legs and in the lower part of the body. This energy flow explains the negative influence of the full

214

moon on the pshycoemotional state of people (especially with a unstable psyche). This also explains classic Veda recommendation to practice fasting on the full moon (in this period the maximum cleansing takes place, because all fluids activate). Observing your state, you can easily notice, that on the full moon it's very difficult to practice hatha, you feel more like meditating, reflecting on something; while at the new moon the body is practically demanding physical training.

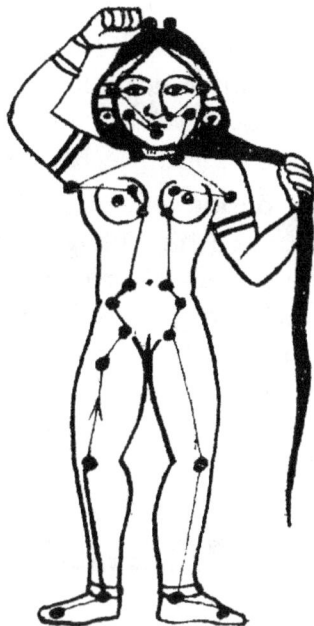

Motion of Energy Flow under the Moon Activity

Figure from Rajasthan miniature of XVIII century

The movement of energy «tide» in our body is shown on the picture. Classic Indian treaties don't specify if the energy movement differs for men and women, but we suppose that it does in the mirror way. For men when the moon is new: the point of maximum influence of the moon is located on the left foot, for women — on the right foot. Then towards the full moon it shifts by the left (right for women) side of the body to come to the head when the moon is full. And for the second phase of the moon, the «growing old», it descends consequently to the right foot for men and to the left foot for women. Thus when the moon is growing, the «high tide» is on the «taking» side, activating functions of energy inflow. When the moon is decreasing, function of outflow activates and the body starts cleansing itself. This rule can be used this way: practices aiming to reinforce, develop chakra (in all senses — from spiritual up to simple muscle training) are better when the moon is growing, while cleansing is better at the descending moon.

Interesting to notice, that these principles are used in phytotherapy. Here is one citation.

«So by this moment passes exactly a half of moon cycle. Then the moon, going around, decreases and is passing chakras in the reverse order. Knowing that chakras are seven and the moon cycle is 28 days, it's easy to count, that every chakra has two days of the moon cycle at the growing moon (the period of energy inflow) and two days at the decreasing moon (period of energy outflow).

Plants, gathered in the respective periods of the moon make the same effect on chakra. For example, bear's foot with blue flowers, picked up in the 11th and 12th days of the moon cycle attracts energy to Ajna; and gathered in 17th and 18th days on the contrary favours the outflow.

In other words, to cleanse the 6th charka from the negative energy the sick person should take broths and infusions of bear foot with blue flowers (plants of the family Aconitum), gathered on the 17th and 18th days of the moon cycle; and to compensate the energy on Ajna — infusions of bear foot, gathered on the 11th and 12th days of the cycle.

A clinical example: thyroiditis, accompanied with the decreased function of thyroid have to be treated by giving the blue-flower bear foot, gathered on the 11th and 12th days of the moon cycle, while the acute laryngitis and thyreotoxicosis — by the same bear foot, gathered on the 17th and the 18th days.

Yellow-flower bear foot the same as the immortelle, dandelion, greater celandine and others have energy activity with Manipura (third chakra), responsible for all the complex of digesting organs, the system of protein synthesis and detoxication. This kind of bear boot should be gathered on the 5-6th and on the 23-24th day of the moon calendar. Chronic hypoacid gastritis, biliary dyskinesia by a hypotonic method are treated by the yellow bear foot of the first period of gathering, while the ulcer disease of duodenum and acute hepatitis — by the gathering of the second period».

Other biological rhythms in the body

A person has a quite complicated system of biological rhythms. Some of them are well-known and even advertised (like so-called «intellectual», «emotional» and «physical» rhythms in every mobile phone — although this information is very doubtful). Other rhythms are little known and not studied at all. Yoga believes that the most important to know is our circadian rhythm. Individual day differs from the real one: outside it can be evening, while by your individual clock it's still morning. Some astrologists believe that the individual midnight depends on the time of birth, but I can't check this information.

In the same manner is built the individual annual rhythm. Summer is individual — i.e. the most activity season is the one, opposite to the season of your birth. Consequently the individual spring is a period of creativity and autumn is a period of summing up.

Chinese medicine also describes the day rhythm, related to the energy movement by our system of meridians. Every one of our 12 channels is on its peak and in its lowest point for 2 hours a day. Organs, related to the channel are the most vulnerable in the moment of decrease. It is when they should be pumped up with energy.

www.ingramcontent.com/pod-product-compliance
Lightning Source LLC
Chambersburg PA
CBHW080621030426
42336CB00018B/3040